THREE ON THE

EDGE

BANTAM BOOKS

NEW YORK TORONTO LONDON

SYDNEY AUCKLAND

THREE ON THE
EDGE

THE STORIES OF ORDINARY AMERICAN FAMILIES

IN SEARCH OF A MEDICAL MIRACLE

JOHN KELLY

THREE ON THE EDGE

A Bantam Book / January 1999

BOOK DESIGN BY DANA LEIGH TREGLIA.

Library of Congress Cataloging-in-Publication Data
Kelly, John, 1945–
Three on the edge / John Kelly.
p.   cm.
ISBN 0-553-10113-7
1. Clinical trials—Patients—United States—Biography.   2. Drugs—Testing.
3. Protolytic enzyme inhibitors—Testing.   4. AIDS (Disease)—Patients—United
States—Biography.   5. Osteosarcoma—Patients—United States—Biography.
6. Breast—Cancer—Patients—United States—Biography.   7. Antineoplastic
agents—Testing.   I. Title
R853.C55K44   1999
615.5'8'0287—dc21   98-25948
CIP

Published simultaneously in the United States and Canada

Bantam Books are published by Bantam Books, a division of Random
House, Inc. Its trademark, consisting of the words "Bantam Books" and the
portrayal of a rooster, is Registered in U.S. Patent and Trademark Office and
in other countries. Marca Registrada. Bantam Books, 1540 Broadway,
New York, New York 10036.

PRINTED IN THE UNITED STATES OF AMERICA

BVG   10   9   8   7   6   5   4   3   2   1

To Eleanor Blake Kelly and

Sheila Weller Kelly

Author's Note

The people and stories portrayed in this book are all real; however, the names and some identifying characteristics of the trial subjects and their families have been changed in most instances. Where noted in the text, the names of some of the physicians and researchers have also been changed.

CONTENTS

INTRODUCTION

1

EDWARD IN
WINTER

13

ROMY'S
KNEE

111

JULIE AND HER
SISTERS

209

AFTERWORD

307

ACKNOWLEDGMENTS

310

INTRODUCTION

In the early summer of 1994, *The New York Times* ran a story about an AIDS drug that I had not heard of before. It was called a protease inhibitor, and according to the *Times*, it had performed extremely well in a new Bellevue Hospital study. AIDS patients live or die by their T cell counts—a measure of HIV activity in the body—and the inhibitor had boosted counts in the Bellevue study by an average of one hundred points. "I have risen from the dead," one ecstatic subject proclaimed to the *Times*. "I feel like Lazarus." The man's elation leaped off the page at me.

What a remarkable experience, I thought—to believe your death preordained, then to be saved by a new medicine. But I also wondered how saved the man really was. After all, the miracle at Bellevue had been a very small miracle. Only thirty or so people had participated in the study, and the study itself was very preliminary. Dozens of promising new AIDS drugs had ended up being outsmarted by wily HIV. The protease inhibitor could easily turn out to be another failure.

A few weeks later, I met with Dr. Roy (Trip) Gulick, the codirector of the study. Trip Gulick was young—in his early thirties—and very excited about the results, though he was trying hard not to show it. "Certainly, we won't know anything conclusive until we do a larger study," he told me. "But I think this drug could turn out to be different. I think we may have something that could change the prognosis for AIDS."

"You mean, cure it?" I asked.

"No, not cure," Dr. Gulick said, "but with the protease inhibitor we might be able to make AIDS a manageable disease like diabetes or heart disease. People won't have to die from it anymore."

Even slightly amended, this claim astonished me. Dr. Gulick's cluttered little office in rundown Bellevue seemed the most unlikely of places to dream of altering the course of an incurable disease—a disease that had killed nearly 50,000 Americans the year before, 8,000 in New York City alone.

Dr. Gulick said that Merck, the company that made the protease inhibitor, was planning to do a larger and more definitive study in the spring of 1995, one that would employ the inhibitor in a new way; in the new trial, it would be combined with two other drugs rather than used alone, as it had been in the first study. He invited me to become an observer. "You could follow one of our subjects," he said.

The offer appealed to me; though very brief, my one other encounter with a clinical trial had left a deep impression on me. In 1992, a close friend had asked me to accompany her and her husband to what would be the most important interview of her life. A few weeks earlier, she had been diagnosed with an inoperable brain tumor. The interview was for admission to a new clinical trial; according to my friend's oncologist, the treatment being tested in the study, borum capture therapy, was the only thing that might be able to help her. It was, quite literally, her last hope. Since I had written extensively on medicine, she wanted me to come along.

Two images from that interview haunted me for weeks. The first was the expression on the neurologist's face when he told my friend that her tumor was too big to qualify for the study. It was the first time

I had ever seen anyone manage to look both sad and detached at the same time. The other was the woman I saw sitting in the waiting room after the interview. She had gotten into the trial. I knew that, because her husband was filling out an admission form for her as I walked out of the neurologist's office.

"They want to know what your first symptom was," I heard him say. "It was double vision, wasn't it?"

The woman shook her head. "No, the headache." The woman paused. "The double vision didn't start until Marie's wedding. Remember?"

"Yes," her husband said, his voice suddenly very soft. "I remember."

Over the next few weeks, I spent a lot of time thinking about this sweet-faced, frightened-looking woman. I wondered about her headache and about what had happened to her at Marie's wedding. I also wondered what was going to happen to her now, in the borum capture trial.

A malignant brain tumor—the price of admission to the study—is almost always fatal. The woman's life—and her husband's, too—would now narrow down to this one unproven and highly risky treatment, in this one clinical trial. For the next six months, the trial would be the focal point of this couple's existence. What would it be like to be in a situation such as that? A situation where the outcomes are so unrelievedly stark—life or death, no in between—and where every moment that passes without a miracle makes it that much less likely that a miracle will happen and save you. How do ordinary people—people like the woman and her husband—function in such an extreme and terrible circumstance? How do they find ways to cope—and how do they find ways to hope?

I also wondered about the neurologist who had disqualified my friend from the study. "I'm sorry," he had told her, "but admission is limited to patients with tumors three centimeters and under; your tumor is three point three centimeters." The decision had struck me as awful: to take away a person's last chance at life because her tumor was a fraction of a fraction of an inch too large. I knew that the neurologist had no alternative; the trial's rules, not he, dictated who got in. Still, he was a human being and he knew what his no meant. What was it like to do what he had done, day in and day out? To say no to people who need a yes, in order to have any kind of chance at life? What did that kind of responsibility do to you after a while?

Eventually these questions began to form into an idea for a book. I thought the experiences of people in a high-stakes trial—a trial for which the likely outcome was life or death—would make a compelling and moving human story and also a story with a universal resonance, since serious illness is something that befalls us all, either directly or when someone close to us becomes ill. By exploring what people are capable of in a moment of supreme crisis, we might learn what we, too, are capable of.

The clinical trial—the workshop of research medicine—would also be a good place to explore what is involved in the creation of new therapies for serious illnesses: to examine the insights and ideas that lead to new drugs and drug combinations, to look at how ideas are fashioned into concrete treatments, and to assess how much progress is being made against common killer diseases.

Dr. Gulick's invitation gave me the one thing I lacked: an organizational plan. I would use a group of personal stories—stories of people I had followed through a clinical trial—to explore the human and scientific side of the most dramatic branch of research medicine.

More than a thousand clinical trials* are conducted annually in the United States. So my first task was to select three studies that would be interesting and significant. I used two criteria for my selections: The trial had to involve a therapy for a common serious illness, and the illness had to be one for which successful treatments were either totally or largely lacking.

---

*No public or private agency tracks the number of clinical trials done each year, so it is impossible to come up with an exact number.

AIDS met both criteria, so I accepted Dr. Gulick's invitation to follow a patient in the new protease inhibitor trial. I was still skeptical about how effective the inhibitor would turn out to be, but I knew that if the drug performed to Dr. Gulick's expectations, it would signal the arrival of a true medical miracle.

The other disease that met my two criteria was cancer. While the death rate from heart disease, the leading killer of Americans, has fallen by almost a third over the past generation, the overall death rate for cancer today is only slightly better than it was in the 1950s. There are a number of reasons for this, but paramount among them is the current state of cancer treatment.

Chemotherapy, oncology's main weapon, has had some stunning successes against individual cancers. But overall, its impact on the disease has been limited. Furthermore, most chemotherapeutic agents are highly toxic. They do terrible things to the human body. They can damage the heart, liver, kidneys, and other vital organs, and they almost always cause debilitating quality-of-life side effects, such as baldness, chronic nausea, fatigue, and bloating.

The two cancer trials I elected to follow both tested medications that, in one way or another, addressed the problems and limitations of chemotherapy. The first trial was conducted a few blocks away from Bellevue at New York University Medical Center; it was testing a new treatment for osteosarcoma, a form of bone cancer that strikes children between the ages of twelve and eighteen. MTP—muramyl tripeptide phosphatidyl ethanolamine—is designed to stop the leading cause of death in OS. Osteosarcoma patients usually die, not from the cancer in their bones, but from the cancer that metastasizes to the lungs; there, the disease quite literally suffocates the child to death. While any agent that could save a youngster from such a terrible death would be important in and of itself, MTP, part of a new generation of non-chemo cancer drugs, also seemed significant for another reason: It worked not by pouring toxic chemicals on cancer cells, but naturally, by enhancing the body's natural cancer-fighting abilities. A success in the NYU trial would not only save many young lives, it could change the way many common adult cancers are treated, too.

The other study I selected for the book was a breast cancer trial at Fox Chase Cancer Center in Philadelphia. Breast cancer is the second leading cause of cancer death among women. Every year, 186,000 women develop breast cancer and 46,000 die from it—a death rate roughly equivalent to the loss of a small city every year. What interested me about the Fox Chase trial is that it was asking an entirely new—and surprising—question about breast cancer and chemotherapy: Maybe the problem with chemo is not that it does not work very well but that we use it the wrong way. The Fox Chase study employed two veteran chemotherapeutic agents, Adriamycin and Cytoxan, but in a radically new manner.

If the strategy worked, it, like MTP, would also change the way many cancers are treated.

My next task was to select a person to follow in each trial.

I began at Bellevue. In April 1995, I spent a week interviewing subjects at the hospital. But the person I finally selected, Edward Sandisfield, refused to meet with me at first. "I'm not right for you," Edward said when I called to arrange an interview. "You want one of those pretty young men with a rage to live. I'm not pretty anymore and I have no rage to live. I have accepted my fate."

I was intrigued. Edward's words were ironic and rueful, but the voice speaking them was neither; it was formal and reserved. If I had to guess, I would say that Edward was a business executive or perhaps a professional man—a lawyer, doctor, or professor.

"I really don't think there is any point in our meeting, Mr. Kelly."

Trip Gulick had warned me to expect wariness at first. Edward was very curious about my book, but also very private. I asked him if I could call again anyway. "Maybe we could talk a little more on the phone," I said.

There was a pause. "All right, if you wish." This time the formal voice was a little warmer.

Three weeks later, I finally coaxed Edward into a face-to-face meeting at Bellevue.

"See, I'm too old for you," he said when Trip Gulick introduced us.

I imagined that Edward had once been quite handsome. He had a high, noble forehead, fine reddish-brown hair, perfectly even features, and the most immaculate white teeth I had ever seen. But six years of living with HIV had taken its toll; the handsome face had become hollowed out, blotchy, and vaguely ill-looking. But the body below the face was still young; it was also clad in young man's clothes: a yellow T-shirt, snug-fitting jeans, and work boots.

"How old are you?" I asked.

"Fifty-four. Quite ancient." Edward's voice remained formal.

He was an interesting puzzle; a rich man who always felt poor, a conscientious man who could behave recklessly, a contentious man who craved friendship, a kind man who could be cruel, and ultimately, a dying man who refused to die. Edward claimed to be tired of life, but I had never met anyone who fought as tenaciously as he to hang on to it.

It would take me a year to discover all of this about him, but I already knew that spring morning at Bellevue that there was something special about Edward, some spark of toughness in him.

My introduction to Romy Hochman, the fourteen-year-old I followed through the MTP study, was arranged by Dr. Aaron Rausen, Romy's physician and a leading expert on osteosarcoma.

Dr. Rausen told me that he had three patients in the new NYU MTP trial: a seventeen-year-old from Staten Island, a twelve-year-old from New Jersey, and Romy, whom Dr. Rausen described as "the daughter of the Bagel King and a Beverly Hills antiques dealer." I was curious about the mother's Beverly Hills address. The Hochmans were divorced, I knew, but I had assumed that Romy, who was from Smith-town, Long Island, lived with her mother. It was unusual for a woman to live a continent apart from her child.

I told Dr. Rausen that I would like to meet the Hochmans.

Four days later, I made my first visit to a place that would assume an almost mystical significance in my mind over the next year—the ninth floor of NYU Medical Center, the pediatric oncology unit. Admitted only a month earlier, Romy already had the ninth-floor look. She was pale and gaunt and very thin and bald. I had been expecting that, but I had also been expecting something else—anger. The labels "Bagel King" and "Beverly Hills antiques dealer" suggested privilege, and I thought that a child of privilege would be especially outraged at a hor-rible injustice like cancer. But I could see no anger in Romy. I thought I saw sadness and resignation, but I was not even sure of that. Romy had a personality that was opaque in ways that went beyond a fourteen-year-old's normal shyness with a stranger.

As we were talking, a very pretty, stylishly dressed blond woman came into the room carrying a pizza.

"This is the clinical trials guy," Romy said, introducing me.

The woman put the pizza down on a chair and smiled. "Hi, Mr. Clinical Trials Guy, I'm Romy's mother, Pam Hochman."

A week later in the medical center courtyard, Pam asked me how much I knew about her.

I told her what Dr. Rausen had told me.

"That's all he said? That I have an antiques store in Beverly Hills?"

I nodded.

I could see Pam thinking. "He didn't say anything about anything else?"

"No," I said.

Pam paused again. "I've been wondering how much I should tell you about myself." Then she let out a deep sigh and told me everything. She said that a drug addiction, begun in college, had spun out of control six years earlier and cost her everything: her marriage, her child (who had elected to live with her father), and very nearly her life. "I spent three years in rehabilitation after the divorce. Then I moved to L.A. and started to put my life back together."

On this chilly October afternoon, the courtyard was empty except for the two of us and a maintenance man, emptying the trash cans into a cart. Pam stared at him for a moment, then turned back to me. "I promised myself that when I was all right again, I would ask Romy to come and live with me. And we're going to. I'm going to see her through this, and when it's over I'm going to take her home with me."

I had come to Romy's room looking for a story of physical healing but I found a story of a different kind of healing there, too.

Cancer is often depicted as an unpredictable, undisciplined disease; the favorite metaphor of medical writers is a rampaging, voracious adolescent. But in Julie Mackey Conte's family, cancer has always behaved like a model citizen. In Julie's family, cancer has removed all the anxious and puzzling guesswork about when or whom it will strike, or what form it will take; the disease always appears as breast cancer, it always strikes at age thirty-four, and it always occurs after the birth of a child. This pattern has repeated itself three times now. With Julie's mother, with Julie's older sister, Jennifer, and now with Julie herself.

When we met four months after Julie's diagnosis, she was still reeling. "None of it feels real to me yet," she said.

On the drive from Philadelphia to Julie's comfortable hilltop home in bucolic Newtown, Pennsylvania, Eric Rosenthal, the director of public affairs at Fox Chase Cancer Center, had given me a brief description of her. He said that Julie was thirty-four, married, had two children, and worked at a local hospital. Eric also said that Julie had an excellent prognosis. Her breast cancer was early stage, and three-quarters of women with early stage disease were still alive ten years later.

Julie was the wrong kind of patient for me, I thought. I was looking for someone who was more seriously ill. But in Julie's family, it turned out that cancer's idiosyncrasies extended to prognosis. During the interview, she said that her mother and sister also had been diagnosed with early stage disease; both were dead within three years.

As Julie and I talked, her eight-month-old son, Mark, kicked in his playpen; Julie's other child, two-year-old Brittany, sat on the other side of the living room watching a videotape of *The Lion King*.

"Do you have any other sisters?" I asked.

"Three," Julie said. "My older sister is thirty-six and my younger sisters are thirty-two and thirty. They're worried about me, but they're worried about themselves, too."

I had wanted to tell a woman's story in the book, and Julie's story seemed preeminently that. There was the nature of her illness, her three sisters, her daughter, and additionally, there was her oncologist, Lori Goldstein, who was the director of the Fox Chase trial. I thought it would be interesting and important to see how research medicine is conducted on a woman-to-woman basis.

Over the year I followed Julie and Romy and Edward, I became a vicarious patient. I sat in on trial interviews and exams, watched my subjects being scanned and X-rayed, saw tubes inserted and removed, saw blood pumped out and chemotherapy pumped in. I read their treatment schedules. I sat with them in hospital cafeterias on summer afternoons, and in infusion rooms on cold winter mornings. I laughed and cried with them and prayed for them. I talked to their friends and spouses and lovers and physicians. I learned what it was like to live with death constantly on your shoulder. And I witnessed victory and defeat—in one case, terrible defeat.

My year of living as a vicarious patient ended in the spring of 1996 when the last of the three studies, the protease inhibitor trial at Bellevue, ended. Between the spring of 1995 and the spring of 1996, I had spent approximately 200 hours with my three subjects, and at the end of that time, I found myself thinking differently about three things.

I had begun the book, in part, to learn how people hope in a nearly hopeless situation, how they sustain themselves when there is no beach or blue sky or Barbara Walters to do a voice-over—just the open mouth of a C/T scan or the silent drip of Adriamycin going from IV bag to tube to vein.

I found that for my three patients, as I suspect for most people caught in a prolonged medical crisis, hope functioned largely on an unconscious level. Romy, Edward, and Julie each had moments of elation, moments when they were sure that everything would come out right, no matter what the doctors and the numbers said. But the day-to-day hope that sustained them was very different. It was a grim, workmanlike emotion, very subtle and tough; it could stand up to almost any kind of bad news and function in any setting; it could also be a terrible bully when it had to be. There were times when I'm sure Edward and Romy wanted to let go, to give up. But even when they wanted hope to shut up and go away, it would not; it would stay and wheedle and bargain and cajole; it would insist that they go on.

I also learned something about the power of human relationships from my three patients. I saw how physically sustaining love could be. Romy, I am convinced, would not have survived the OS or the MTP trial without Pam or her father, Jack—nor would Julie have survived breast cancer without her large and loving family. But I also found that human relationships sustain for other reasons. The pleasure Edward took in driving everyone around him (including me) crazy was also a physical restorative. Edward always felt more energetic and involved in life on days when he was planning to stick a rocket in someone's ear. After a year of watching Julie and Romy and Edward, I have come to believe that human beings can stand up to anything—*anything*—as long as they do not have to stand up to it alone.

I also think there is a lesson to be drawn from these three stories, from who got their miracle and who did not, from who was saved and who was not. The lesson is about the workings of grace and good fortune in life and whether they occur randomly, are distributed on the basis of worthiness, or whether, in the end, we make our own good fortune, our own miracles. But I leave it to the reader to decide what the lesson is.

EDWARD IN WINTER

CHAPTER ONE

ONE UNSEASONABLY COOL MORNING IN MAY 1989, EDWARD SANDIS-field stopped in front of the Golden Apple, a greengrocer on the corner of First Avenue and Thirty-second Street, and began to cry. Edward's tears seemed to upset the moonfaced Korean man hosing down the flower racks in front of the store. He stared at Edward for a moment, then turned off the hose and began to walk back toward the store's entrance. At the door, he stopped suddenly and looked over his shoulder. This time his gaze was more contemptuous than hostile. Edward ✕ flushed. God, what a lovely sight he must make! Sweaty, in running shorts, and weeping. Edward the Beautiful!

A few other things about that May morning also remain vivid to Edward: He remembers waking up around six with a nervous stomach and lying in bed listening to the rumble of the M15 bus on sleepy Seventy-eighth Street below and he remembers the dazzling vista that greeted him when he went out to the terrace around seven with his coffee: morning light, glorious and golden, dancing on windows all the way up Seventy-eighth to the park.

Edward also recalls exactly where he was when his plan for this day began to unravel. The morning he learned that his HIV test was scheduled for May twenty-third, Edward decided that he would combine the test with some daily thing in his life to make it seem like less of an Event. The thing he decided on was running. Instead of his usual two laps around the Central Park reservoir, on the twenty-third he would jog down to the Department of Health testing facility on Twenty-sixth Street from his apartment on East Seventy-eighth Street.

At first the plan worked well. The tingle of cool spring air against his face; the soft clip-clop of his footfalls on the early morning sidewalk; the canopy of freshly bloomed trees overhead—the sights and sounds of this gorgeous spring morning all worked their magic. Turning onto First Avenue, Edward felt centered, calm, and prepared.

But at Forty-seventh Street, the strategy started to unravel. Edward felt his eyes misting up; at Thirty-second Street in front of the Golden Apple, he was crying so hard he had to stop. The enormity of the day, of what he was about to do, of the change his life was about to take—all the big, awful things Edward had planned so meticulously to avoid thinking about—finally overwhelmed him.

Edward continued crying until he noticed the greengrocer's wife staring at him through the plate-glass window. She was making a waving motion with the back of her hand as if she were trying to shoo him away. Edward stared at her for a moment, then tried to resume his jog, but he had no heart left; a block later, he began to walk. At Twenty-sixth and First, he stopped in front of a four-story brick building. Decades of gas fumes and pigeon droppings had turned the white façade a strange gray-yellow-green color. As he removed the appointment card from his fanny pack, Edward examined the building.

The windows were covered with heavy iron gates; inside, he could see a policeman standing behind the revolving door. The place looked like a prison. Edward supposed it was.

Going through the revolving door, he touched the sore on his forehead. Ouch, it still hurt. Gently, he touched it again. This time, a few pieces of dead skin fell off on his fingertips.

Too much sun was Edward's first thought when he noticed the sore a month ago on a flight from Acapulco to L.A. But the dermatologist in Los Angeles said no; sun was not the problem. The configuration of the sore was unique to herpes zoster. Edward nodded, but didn't ask any questions; he was already familiar with herpes zoster. Just before he left for Mexico, the GMHC (Gay Men's Health Crisis) *Bulletin* had run an article on the skin condition. According to the piece, herpes zoster (popularly known as shingles) was a common first sign of HIV infection.

Edward walked to the elevator, where a muscular young man in a T-shirt, snug-fitting jeans, and work boots smiled at him. Just as Edward was about to smile back, the elevator doors snapped open; the young man disappeared into a knot of clamoring bodies. Edward waited until the elevator was full, then stepped in and pressed three.

Four years earlier, Edward would have found his presence in this elevator inconceivable. Well into the mid-1980s, he dismissed AIDS as a disease of "others," of street hustlers, male prostitutes, drug addicts. People like him did not get infected—people who owned second homes in the Hamptons, vacationed in Aspen and Gstaad, who antiqued on weekends, collected art; people who cooked gourmet meals for one another. But Jack Scarf had shattered that illusion. One night in 1987, Corky Wilcox, Jack's lover and an old friend of Edward's, had called, frantic. Corky had just found Jack asleep on the living room couch in a pool of perspiration.

"He's having a night sweat," Corky said. "You know what that means, Edward. He's infected and if he's infected I must be, too." Edward kept his own voice even and unemotional. But after he hung up, a new thought burst into his mind; he had had just as many lovers as Corky and Jack. Maybe he was infected, too.

An elbow pressed into his back. Edward was pushed against the elevator doors. The steel felt cold against his damp T-shirt. Edward moved back. Shit. The elbow knifed into his shoulder blades again. Edward was about to confront his tormentor when the doors opened suddenly and he was thrust into a large hallway, which was even dirtier than the outside of the building. Cigarette butts, gum wrappers, empty bottles, and cups littered the floor. The smell of stale smoke, human sweat, and coffee hung over everything. A dozen or so people, most of them men, were sitting on the benches along the corridor. No one looked up when Edward walked by.

"Do you have a number, sir?" the clerk at the registration desk asked.

Edward shook his head.

The clerk punched a code into the computer behind the desk, then looked at Edward. "You are number seven twenty-eight, sir." He handed Edward a pamphlet and told him he would be required to see a counselor before the test.

"How long is the wait?"

The clerk smiled. "Oh, soon, sir, very soon." He was Indian and his accent made the reassurance sound almost melodic.

The bench at the far end of the hall was empty except for an obese, bald-headed man in matching black leather vest, pants, and motorcycle boots. Edward walked over, sat down next to him, and opened the Department of Health pamphlet; it reiterated what a caseworker had told him on the phone a week earlier: at DOH testing facilities, clients were identified by number only; the use of names was forbidden, even in DOH files. To Edward, this promise more than made up for the dirt and the crowds.

A whining sound rose above the din in the hall. Someone was crying. Edward had been warned about breakdowns. "Some people sob and yell when they get their results," a friend had told him. "DOH can get very ugly. You better prepare yourself." Edward put the booklet down and scanned the benches again; they were full of the kind of people he had spent his life trying to get away from.

"Owwwwwwwww." The sob exploded into a wail, then stopped. A

door opened near the registration desk and a thin, tentative-looking young man walked out. He was about twenty-one or twenty-two, and had a long, narrow face and a wispy Custer-style blond goatee. The skin beneath his eyes was very red. The young man seemed reluctant to move. He stood trembling in the doorway until a tall, slim young woman in a calf-length dress and hoop earrings appeared from inside the office. She whispered something to the young man, then put her arm around him and walked him to the elevator.

"Remember, call me," Edward heard her say when the elevator arrived. The young man nodded, then stepped inside. Edward felt relieved when the elevator doors shut.

A few minutes later, the young woman reappeared in the hall. She looked at the card in her hand, then called, "Seven twenty-eight." Edward's number.

"My name is Sarah," she said when he stood up, "and you are"— she looked at the card again—"you are seven twenty-eight. Please." She gestured toward the open door.

Her office was small and dark except for a single shaft of sunlight; the light spilled over plants and pictures on the windowsill and onto a chair in the center of the room. Edward felt as if he had slipped inside a chocolate bar with a golden caramel center. He sat in the chair, then pushed it back into the shade. The spring sun felt hot against his naked legs. Above the desk, specks of dust danced in the light.

"So," the young woman said, removing a piece of paper from a folder, "how are you today, seven twenty-eight?" Edward was surprised at how pretty she was. Under the fluorescent lights in the hall, she had looked washed out. The *Masterpiece Theatre* gold-and-mahogany tones in here flattered her.

"Are you nervous? It's okay. Most of my visitors are."

"No," Edward lied. Behind him, he could hear the low hum of a humidifier. It muffled the din in the hall.

The young woman smiled. "Good, don't be. I'm here to be your friend."

Edward felt his anxiety draining away. He had been expecting a bureaucrat. This young woman, Sarah, was a wonderful surprise; she was warm and empathic. Maybe she was a good omen.

"There are some questions I'd like to ask you," Sarah said. "You don't have to answer any of them, but the more we know about HIV, the more we can do to help people."

She removed a piece of paper from a folder, picked up a pencil, then smiled at Edward. "So tell me about yourself."

Edward said he was forty-eight, single, and a self-employed marketing consultant, who divided his time between New York and Miami. He owned an apartment on East Seventy-eighth Street, another in South Beach.

"What about family?" Sarah asked.

Edward told her he had two brothers, one older, one younger; they lived in Seattle. His mother lived there, too.

Sarah made a note in the file, then looked up. "Does your family know you are here today? About the test?"

"No," Edward said.

Edward's relationship with his family was complex. Sometimes, when pressed, he would say that his mother, Evelyn, had an "intuitive knowledge" of his homosexuality, that the mothers of gay men always knew the truth on some level. But other times Edward would insist that Evelyn had absolutely no idea he was gay. No one in his family did.

Edward laughed ruefully when Sarah asked him about lovers.

"I take it that's a no, seven twenty-eight?"

"A definite, emphatic no," Edward said.

Edward hadn't had a regular lover since . . . when? Since Colin walked out on him in . . . 1983? Edward's other former lovers were either dead or dying. Recently, looking through his address book, Edward found every fourth or fifth name Xed out. Early on, when people first started to die, he used to put a little notation next to each crossed-out name, some little thought about the person, but there were so many people dying now, he just crossed the names out. Todd Clarke's was the latest to be Xed out. Todd had died three months ago, on February seventh. Edward remembered the date because he had just arrived in Saint Moritz for a two-week skiing vacation when he got a call from half a world away telling him that his old lover had passed away.

"Which method of exposure might have brought you into contact with the HIV virus?" Sarah asked. "HIV drug use, blood transfusion, or sexual contact?"

"Sexual contact," Edward said.

"Heterosexual or homosexual?"

"Homosexual."

Edward could still remember the name of his first lover, Michael Jefferies, and where they met—the roof of the Seattle YMCA. One steamy August afternoon in 1960 the tall, doe-eyed Jefferies, a Northwest Airlines pilot, approached nineteen-year-old Edward while he was sunbathing. "Would you like to have dinner with me?" Jefferies asked in a silky baritone. The next morning, Edward felt shamed and frightened by the things he and Jeffries had done, but also thrilled, thrilled almost beyond words.

Sarah put down the pencil. She suddenly looked very somber.

"Do you think you're positive?"

Edward hesitated for a moment. "Yes," he said finally; his intuition told him that he was.

"What will you do if you are?"

"I don't know," Edward said. "It's like asking me what I would do if I lived on Mars. I don't have any reference points yet. I'll have to live with the virus for a while." He paused again. "I suppose it won't do much for my love life, though, being infected? There isn't much of a market for forty-eight-year-olds as it is. God knows what the market will be for an HIV-positive forty-eight-year-old."

Ten days later, in the same hall, Sarah called Edward's number again. She smiled when he stood up. That was a good omen, Edward thought—Sarah's smile—and he noticed that the smile was particularly bright this morning. Another good omen. But seeing her again, rather than another counselor; something told Edward that was not a good sign.

This time, there were no preliminaries. Sarah did not exactly rush Edward, but she didn't make small talk either. She was businesslike. As soon as the two of them were seated she said, "I'm afraid your intuition was right, seven twenty-eight."

"I'm positive?" Edward asked.

"Yes, the test indicates you are."

Later Edward would say that at that moment, he slipped into a parallel universe. Everything in this new universe was exactly the same. Sarah was the same, the chair he was sitting in was the same. The streaks of rain on the window, the honking sounds of traffic floating up from the street below. But life in this parallel universe was also utterly different. It was starker, more severe, more unforgiving, and colder. Especially colder. No fires of expectation warmed you here.

When Sarah asked what he planned to do, Edward got annoyed. "I told you last week, I don't know. I'll have to live with this thing for a while."

Edward had misunderstood her, Sarah said. She did not mean what was he going to do six months from now. She meant what was he going to do now, today, when he left this office. "Some people get suicidal when they receive their test results," she said. "I want to know you'll be all right today. I need to know that you'll have a support system around you."

Edward said he had a doctor's appointment that afternoon, a dinner date in the evening.

Sarah wrote the information down and handed Edward an envelope with the number 728 written on the front. The five-by-eight card inside contained Edward's test results.

The hall was much less crowded today. There were only about a half dozen people sitting on the benches. As he walked to the elevator,

Edward noticed a sign above one of the benches. GHMC was throwing a Body Positive Tea Dance at its headquarters on Twenty-second Street this coming Sunday. EVERYONE'S INVITED!!! the sign said.

Edward tried to imagine a room full of HIV-positive men dancing, but couldn't. Life on Mars, he thought, and pressed the elevator button.

CHAPTER TWO

ONCE, WHEN HE WAS FIVE YEARS OLD, EDWARD LEAPED UP ONTO A living-room chair and smashed an ashtray into his father's skull. The blow, which sprayed tiny flecks of blood all over Edward's face and arms, stunned Stephen Sandisfield; his hand dropped from his wife's head and he slumped to the living room floor, howling in pain. For that one brief moment, five-year-old Edward felt in control of the crazy, unpredictable universe around him.

Edward was born on August 18, 1941, in Stroudsburg, Pennsylvania, a small town near the Delaware Water Gap. But a year later the Sandisfields moved east to New Jersey, where Stephen, an unemployed laborer, found war work at a GM factory. Edward remembers that his father had a thin, hard-bitten face and a nasty temper when he drank, but that's about all he remembers. The last time he saw Stephen Sandisfield was on the morning of April 11, 1947. An hour after Stephen left for work, Evelyn told Edward and his big brother, Tom, to go upstairs and pack; the three of them were leaving for Washington State on the noon train. They were going to live with Evelyn's mother, GeGe.

Edward's earliest memory of his mother is of the
ing on a street corner in East Orange on a wind
watching a big black Chevrolet circle around and
ward guesses he was about five at the time, and he
the third pass around the block, the Chevrolet sto
man in a Dick Tracy hat and a white shirt got ou
young to understand what the man said, but he rec
laughed and smiled at the stranger.

When he was nine, there was a similar incident
tion. As Edward and his mother were walking ou
group of sailors suddenly burst into whistles. By this
old enough to understand what was happening.
whistling because his mother was very pretty. Pictu
disfield taken in the late forties bear out Edward'
show a young woman with a voluptuous figure, and
full of sensuality. But there is also a hint of carelessne
lyn looks like the kind of woman who could be di
man, a few drinks, and a good time. And sometimes

Shortly after the Sandisfields moved back to N
1951, Grandmother GeGe arrived unannounced o
Seattle. The next morning, when Edward came down
and his big brother, Tom, were already dressed; the
the kitchen next to two battered suitcases. Evelyn w
the sink with her arms folded. "Tommy's going to liv
while," she told Edward.

No one explained why Tommy was taken away,
able to figure that out for himself. A few weeks earlie
died of a ruptured appendix because Evelyn, out of e
distraction, had waited nearly a week before calling a
bringing Tommy to Seattle to make sure that never ha

Four years later, GeGe returned to New Jersey;
ward. "I don't know how you could let that man hit
remembers GeGe telling his mother the September m

llect him. The two women were sitting in the Sandisfields' living
, Evelyn in a wing chair by the window, GeGe on the sofa. Edward
crouched under the hall staircase, eavesdropping.

'Lane didn't mean it," Evelyn said. "He just has a bad temper."

Lane is a son of a bitch," GeGe said.

Lane" was Lane B. Hopwell, Evelyn's current lover, a Sinatra-thin
er with dark, oily good looks and glistening jet-black hair. Edward
mbers that Lane was particularly vain about that hair. Even on
ings when Lane was horribly hungover, it would always be slicked
and gleaming when he came downstairs for breakfast. The pecu-
mell of whiskey and cheap hair tonic that used to hang in the
en on those mornings stayed with Edward for a very long time.

ane, like Evelyn's other lovers, was also a nasty drunk. Once in a
ken rage, he snatched a sword from Tom's Civil War collection,
vhacked Edward across the shoulder with the handle. A few years
he attacked Edward again, this time while Edward was wash-
he dinner dishes. But on this occasion, Edward, who was now al-
sixteen, struck back; he turned around and flung a frying pan at
's head.

dward isn't sure how GeGe found out about Lane's attacks.
e his aunt Eunice, his mother's older sister, told her. But he does
mber how relieved he felt that September morning when GeGe
him to go upstairs and pack his things; she was taking him back to
le. Evelyn, who didn't protest when Tommy was taken away from
protested now.

'Please don't take my other boy away," Edward heard her say as he
coming downstairs with his suitcase. She was still sitting in the
chair. But GeGe had moved. She was standing over her daugh-
ow.

'Evelyn," Edward remembers her saying, "I'm sorry, but you're not
be a mother to your boys."

However, six months later, when the newly married Hopwells
d to Seattle, GeGe agreed to let Edward and Tom live with Evelyn

again. The following year, Evelyn had a baby: Edward's half-brother Darryl.

Edward, generally an unsentimental man, is very sentimental about the Seattle gay underground he entered in the early 1960s. After Evelyn and Lane and the dreadful tract house on Mercer Island, the men Edward met in the bars and clubs around Pioneer Square seemed almost magically charming and sophisticated. They knew how to order wine and food, how to talk about art and literature, how to do all the things Edward admired and wanted to learn how to do.

Edward's new friends also liked him. He was a very handsome young man, dark haired with small penetrating blue eyes, a wiry, muscular body, and the most perfect white teeth imaginable. One night, an older man told Edward he had a body like Paul Newman's in *Hud*. The compliment pleased him immensely.

In addition to good looks, Edward also possessed ambition, discipline, intelligence, and a genius for personal reinvention. Once every decade or so for the next thirty years, the old Edward would molt and a new Edward would appear in his place.

The first Edward, the sensual, explosive bad boy of the Seattle gay scene, was replaced within a few years by the smooth, self-assured, corporate Edward. This Edward acquired a Stanford MBA, held a series of increasingly important jobs in Fortune 500 companies—companies where being or appearing gay could destroy a career—and at the relatively young age of thirty-seven, became vice president and marketing director of a large European petroleum company's North American division.

The corporate Edward was an extremely acquisitive creature. He owned a co-op on East Seventy-eighth Street, a house in East Hampton, a condominium in Puerto Vallarta, and a closet full of suits from Barney's.

The last and most imaginative of Edward's creations, the international marketing consultant and sometime playboy, emerged in the 1980s after Edward left the petroleum company. This Edward lived on a different planet from the *Hud*-like sexual desperado. He added an apartment in the newly fashionable South Beach section of Miami to his list of residences, summered in Ramatuelle, a small town outside Saint Tropez, skied in Saint Moritz, and socialized with minor European royalty. He was seen at gallery openings and concerts in Berlin, Amsterdam, Stockholm, and Geneva with a series of young men who were all really the same young man: a blond, blue-eyed Nordic type who spoke English with a charming accent, came from a good family, and was educated at an ancient and prestigious university.

Exactly when this last Edward became infected with HIV is hard to tell. After his best friend Corky Wilcox tested positive in early 1987, Edward, normally extremely health conscious, struck a compromise with his nagging conscience: he would have his T cells monitored—an indirect measure of HIV. However, until the spring of 1989, when the herpes zoster appeared, Edward refused to be tested directly. He says now that he refused because he was afraid; he was sure a positive result would ruin the wonderful life he had built for himself. And he was right; it did.

One night in July 1980, Edward saw a tall, athletically built young man in tan Bermuda shorts and a blue polo shirt walking up the back-porch steps of his home in East Hampton, New York, behind Jack Scarf. Even on the dimly lit porch, Edward could see that Jack's new friend had a pair of shoulders that went on forever. Corky Wilcox also had light brown wavy hair, a big, honking voice, and the weathered, well-bred good looks of a certain kind of Waspy athlete, a country-club golf pro or a weekend yachtsman.

For the next few years, Edward and Corky saw each other only a few times a year. But after Jack got sick, they began to grow close. In the slow, agonizing year of Jack's death, Edward was a model of thoughtfulness and compassion. He called and visited frequently, and when Jack began to die, he accompanied Corky and Jack back to Jack's parents' house in Oklahoma. Sometimes Corky found Edward abrasive, and God knows, Edward was controlling, but he also was funny and smart, and he possessed a weightiness, a certain hard spine of character that Corky found lacking in most of his other friends.

Edward, in his turn, liked Corky's randiness, his wicked sense of fun, and the solidity—the Connecticut Yankee good sense—underneath the playboy exterior. There was also something else he liked about Corky and Corky knew it. "I'm the kind of person Edward would like to be," he told a mutual acquaintance one day. There is a good deal of truth in this observation. Cos Cob, Connecticut, Phillips Exeter Academy, and Yale, a successful family brokerage house, a famous movie-star uncle: Corky possessed the kind of good breeding—the kind of leafy, John Cheever pedigree—that Edward especially admired (though he often reminded himself that in terms of career, he had climbed far higher than Corky and done it with far fewer advantages).

As all long friendships do over the years, Edward and Corky's grew byzantine, dotted with hidden resentments and inadvertencies. They became experts on each other's faults, dished each other endlessly and enthusiastically, yet there remained between them a core of mutual regard and trust. When trouble arose, they usually turned to each other first.

Thus, one morning in October 1994, five years after his HIV test, and three weeks after the appearance of a strange and troubling new symptom, Edward picked up the phone and called Corky.

"Hello. Are you awake?"

Corky looked at the clock on the nightstand next to his bed: 8:00 A.M. Edward, a serious economizer, never called during peak hours. This morning he had saved money twice. An off-hour call on a weekend day.

"Edward, it's Saturday."

"I know what day it is, thank you."

Corky had not spoken to Edward since March. Under the best of circumstances Edward was a high-maintenance friend. But he had outdone even his own hyper-controlling self during an end-of-winter ski trip to Vermont. On Friday, Edward refused to get in the car until Corky agreed to follow his directions to Killington. On Saturday, he made Corky wait until ten o'clock to eat dinner because Edward's gastrointestinal system ran on European time. Finally on Sunday, Corky decided he had had enough; when Edward pointed to a spot in the ski lodge's nearly empty parking lot and said, "Park *there*," Corky turned to him and said, "Edward, this is my fucking car. I'll park it wherever I want to park it."

"How are things in Miami?" Corky asked. "You're getting out aren't you, Edward? You're not sitting alone in that little apartment of yours?"

Corky isn't sure when he first noticed that Edward had begun to let go of life, to isolate himself. He thinks it may have been 1992 or '93. But he does remember what occasioned his concern—a conversation with Avery Goldstein, a mutual friend. Avery, who had just spent a week in South Beach, told Corky that he was worried about Edward. All he did anymore, Avery said, was sit on his terrace, drink gin, talk about his T cells, and complain about how much his doctors and lawyers were charging him.

"Well, yes, Avery's right," Edward conceded a few weeks later when Corky gave him an edited version of this conversation. "I'm not as active as I used to be. But that's because of my reduced financial circumstances." Edward always used his businessman's voice when he talked about money. "You know as well as I do, Corky, if you want to be a player at our age, you need the aphrodisiac of a bank account. And I'm practically broke."

It was, Corky supposed, a leftover from a childhood of near-poverty, but Edward always found a way to reduce every problem in his life to money. He had done it when he was wealthy, and he continued to do it now, when a series of bad investments had reduced him to the New York apartment and the South Beach condo. Six months later, during another conversation, Corky got closer to the truth. Again, Edward pleaded reduced financial circumstances, but this time when Corky pressed him about isolating himself, Edward admitted that money wasn't the only reason he didn't go out anymore.

"You know how HIV neuters you," Edward said. "People run the other way when they hear you're positive. If I stay home I don't have to think about all the things I want but can't have anymore. If I go out to a restaurant or a bar, I do. My old life is all around me . . ." Edward let the rest of the thought speak for itself.

According to another mutual friend, Alan Gillis, who had just come back from Miami, Edward was still sitting on his terrace, except now he was sitting there alone. According to Alan, a few weeks earlier, Edward had had a terrible fight with Martha Bender, a retired teacher who was his last remaining close friend in Miami.

Corky was about to ask Edward about Martha when Michael Stans, Corky's lover, walked into the bedroom looking for his slippers.

"I think they're in there," Corky said, pointing to the bedroom closet.

"What's in there?" Edward asked.

"I'm sorry," Corky said. "I was talking to Michael. He's looking for his slippers."

Edward pictured Michael's wan, pale face. He could not understand what Corky saw in Michael outside of the fact that he was half Corky's age.

Edward got to the point of the call. He had been having gastric distress for the past few weeks. A lot of it.

Corky was surprised. Except for a few minor, transitory symptoms, Edward's health had remained good since his HIV diagnosis.

"When did the distress start?" Corky asked.

"The last week in September," Edward replied. "At first, I thought it was stress. I was in Quebec City with you-know-who that week." Corky smiled. One of Edward's most endearing qualities was his never-ending campaign to improve, to uplift Evelyn Sandisfield. In middle age, he had taken to calling her "Mother," to buying her clothes, to showing her how to eat, to walk and talk—to being her Henry Higgins. But Evelyn had remained stubbornly unimprovable. She still liked Canadian Club neat, olive loaf sandwiches, and men with a Sinatra smile.

Corky asked Edward if he was having distress or pain.

"Pain sometimes."

"Have you seen anyone about it?"

Edward said that he had flown up to New York the previous Thursday to see Don Kotler, a gastroenterologist at St. Luke's–Roosevelt Hospital. "Kotler's pretty sure the distress is HIV related," Edward said. "But nothing showed up on the tests. I want another opinion. I still think it might be stress." Edward asked Corky for the number of his GI specialist at Yale–New Haven Hospital.

Edward never called the gastroenterologist. A few days later, his GI distress mysteriously began to abate, but it was quickly replaced by a new symptom. Shaving one morning in early November, Edward noticed a gauntness in his face. He looked as if he were hollowing out, especially through the cheeks and mouth. He leaned into the bathroom mirror and pinched the skin around his cheeks. The muscle and tissue underneath felt thin and flaccid. Maybe that's why his teeth and eyes had begun to look so prominent lately, Edward thought. Maybe the cheek and jaw muscles that used to frame his face were atrophying. HIV could do that. Edward had seen the virus do it to his old lover Todd Clarke. Toward the end, as his digestive system failed, Todd's facial muscles and tissues wasted away until there was nothing left of his face but two enormous bulging eyes and bone, bone everywhere. Edward leaned into the mirror and pinched the skin around his cheeks again. Could the mysterious indigestion be the first sign of a serious GI system breakdown?

In early December, Edward had another scare. One evening he knocked over a wineglass at dinner. Somehow, he misjudged the glass's position on the table and hit the rim with the back of his hand. Normally, Edward would have dismissed the accident as carelessness, but there had been several similar mishaps lately: one afternoon, a jar of mustard had mysteriously slipped out of his hand, and the day after Corky called, he had had trouble getting an umbrella out of the closet.

Coordination problems can be an early sign of AIDS-related dementia or neurological deterioration. So the night he knocked over the wineglass, Edward decided to conduct an experiment. He picked up the fallen glass, placed it next to his plate, then reached for it again. Edward's thumb and index finger landed securely on the rim. As long as he was paying attention, his coordination seemed fine. Emboldened, Edward decided to repeat the experiment, this time more scientifically. He had read somewhere that shutting your eyes intensifies neurological problems. So this time Edward closed his eyes, then reached for the wineglass. Voilà! His hand landed squarely on the glass again.

Ever since his diagnosis, Edward had treated every new symptom this way. He walked around it, studied it from different angles, ran his hand over its surface, felt its texture. Then he sat down and tried to figure out how to domesticate it, to control it. And up until the early winter of 1994, the technique had worked well. Always or almost always, Edward was able to come up with a credible nonalarming explanation for the changes he noticed in himself. But just after Christmas he finally came face-to-face with a symptom that suggested that all the other little changes he had noticed over the fall—the gauntness, the GI distress, the coordination problems—were related.

T cell count is among the most commonly used gauges of the HIV viral activity in the body. A healthy immune system produces between 500 and 1,500 T cells per microliter of blood; an HIV-affected but still relatively intact immune system, between 300 and 500 T cells per microliter; a seriously impaired system—one capable of producing AIDS-like symptoms—between 200 and 300. T cell counts below 200 indicate the presence of full-blown AIDS. Since 1989, Edward's T cell counts had hovered between 450 and 500: not perfect, but indicative of a certain stability; the body that had been so kind to the young Edward was still being kind to him. It was holding its own against the virus.

But at the end of 1994, Edward's body began to give a little. One morning, a few days after Christmas, Sanford Levinson,* Edward's principal New York doctor, called South Beach. Levinson's high-pitched voice, usually intimate and schmoozy, was crisp and businesslike this morning; he sounded like Richard Simmons in empathy withdrawal.

Edward sensed trouble. "Something wrong, Sandy?" A preemptive strike. Levinson hated the nickname almost as much as Edward hated bad news.

"I have your new count, Edward," Levinson said, refusing to rise to the bait. "I'm afraid your T cells have fallen significantly." In September, Edward's T cell count had been a relatively buoyant 459.

"What does 'significantly' mean?" Edward asked.

"Two sixty-eight," Levinson said.

Edward asked Levinson to repeat the new number.

"Two hundred and sixty-eight, Edward."

"Two hundred and sixty-eight?"

"It could be an aberration, Edward. Why don't we do another test? I'll call a lab down there and make an appointment for you."

Edward said he would be in New York next week.

"Okay. Fine. We'll do it when you come up."

After Levinson hung up, Edward went into the living room and took a folder out of a desk drawer; then he made a drink for himself and walked out to the terrace. Off to the left, near Star Island, a large white Carnival cruise ship was approaching the Miami Harbor channel. Edward stared at it for a moment, then sat down and opened the folder. On top was a copy of his will. Evelyn Sandisfield was listed as sole beneficiary. Should she die first, GMHC would get Edward's two apartments and whatever money and stocks were left. His brothers Tom and Darryl and Darryl's children were not mentioned. Under the

*Pseudonym

legal will was a copy of Edward's living will. It authorized Dr. Sanford Levinson to make medical decisions in the event that Edward became too incapacitated to make them for himself. The third document in the folder, a letter of intent, was addressed to Edward's attorney, Steven Clark. The letter instructed Clark what to tell his family in the event that Edward became too ill to speak for himself.

Edward thought of the arrangement with Clark as an act of charity. He was sparing his mother and brothers, protecting them from worry and pain until the last possible moment. But the arrangement could be interpreted as an act of anger. You have to earn the right to know about another person's private life, and Edward didn't feel that anyone in his family had earned that right. Darryl called him once a year, Tom, once every two, and Evelyn . . . God, Evelyn: He would give her his money, but that was all.

The last item in the folder was a pamphlet; Edward had picked it up in Amsterdam the previous spring. It explained the Dutch government's policy on euthanasia. Edward would have the pamphlet translated now.

That night, Edward had a strange dream. When he woke up the next morning, the only detail he could remember was a single haunting image: himself, a tiny, black, sticklike figure, trudging through a vast, endless, empty snowfield. But gradually, as the day progressed, other details of the dream came back. Edward remembered that a howling bitter wind ripped across the snowfield and on the horizon a thin orange band rose to meet a gray-black sky. Edward also remembered that when he finally reached the horizon and saw that the orange band was really an enormous wall of fire, he thought: If I am lucky the fire will kill me quickly, and if I am not lucky, it will kill me slowly.

CHAPTER THREE

"No, no, you not the boss, I the boss. I decide."

Candy Talcbucon giggled. "You a naughty boy to talk to me like that." Candy had lived in America for fifteen years, but her Filipino accent was still very thick.

Candy giggled again. "You the sweetest talker, you know that." She had been on the phone ten minutes already. Too much time to give to one caller, especially on a morning like this. But this person was hard to say good-bye to; he was funny and charming—an irresistible talker.

It was the day after New Year's 1995 and the AIDS clinical trials unit at Bellevue Hospital in New York City should have been quiet. But a dozen calls had already come in; it had been like this nearly every day since last July, when *The New York Times* ran a front-page story about the unit's successful test of a new anti-AIDS agent, a protease inhibitor called indinavir. Initially the calls were from the tristate area: from New York, Connecticut, and New Jersey. But after a *Nightline* special on the drug in October, calls began coming in from California, Arizona, Toronto, Mexico City, even from Guam. And everyone who called wanted to know the same two things: When was Bellevue going to run a new protease inhibitor study? And could they participate?

In one sense, the torrent of calls was not unusual. Unlike other areas of medicine, where trial subjects are hard to recruit, in HIV people are aggressive in seeking out experimental new therapies. Every day, research centers, pharmaceutical companies, and government laboratories receive hundreds of blind calls about upcoming studies. But the *Times* and *Nightline* stories, which described the protease inhibitor as a new-generation anti-AIDS agent, produced unprecedented interest. No one at the Bellevue unit, a research arm of New York University Medical Center, had seen anything quite like it before. In November, one caller gave the staff a hint of how fierce the competition would be for trial spots in a new indinavir study. He offered Candy $50,000 if she would guarantee him a place in the trial.

Dr. Roy (Trip) Gulick, deputy director of the unit, decided to institute a phone log. The name and telephone number of every caller would be entered in the log; the date of every call would also be recorded. If a new study was organized, the people in the log would be offered spots in the order that they had called. Candy looked at the list now. She was not surprised to find her current caller's name first. Not only had he called earlier than anyone else, he had called more often than anyone else. Twice in October, twice in November, and twice in December.

"You only get one more call this month, Edward."

"You're a terrible woman, Ms. Talcbucon."

Candy asked Edward the temperature in Miami. The question was the opening line in a little piece of shtick the two of them had developed over the months.

"Eighty-three," Edward said, "but it's still early."

Now it was Candy's turn. She would ask Edward what he was going to do today. Edward would say he planned to work on his tan; Candy would respond, "Another tough day at the office"; then the two of them would burst into laughter.

Edward, endlessly charming when he needed to be, had similar phone relationships with Ann Richardson, a trial coordinator at the State University of New York; Joan Sullivan of the University of Miami; and Nancy Steele of the University of North Carolina Medical Center at Raleigh-Durham. Edward called these women regularly to inquire about new studies at their institutions and to swap gossip and information.

Edward also corresponded regularly with several drug company researchers and participated in studies; he had been in an AZT trial when AZT was *the* hot new AIDS drug, and he was currently in a trial of ddI, another hot new AIDS drug, at Columbia-Presbyterian Hospital in New York City. Edward also had created what amounted to a personal medical staff: two doctors in New York, two in Miami, and auxiliary specialists up and down the East Coast.

Often, all the research, the calls and faxes, the flirting—not to mention all the tests and drugs—struck Edward as foolish. He had seen a dozen friends do what he was doing now and the luckiest among them had bought only a few extra months. But whenever Edward thought of surrendering, of letting go, of simply enjoying whatever time and good health he had left, he came up against a force even more implacable than the virus.

Traditionally, the images of hope are gentle, delicate, lovely: a white dove soaring into a limitless blue sky, or a sun-dappled country road on a May afternoon. But Edward's hope was not like these things at all; it was like Edward himself: abrasive, contentious, cunning, single-minded, fearless, controlling, and above all, relentless. Edward's hope cajoled, chided, commanded, pushed, prodded, and nudged. Hope exhausted Edward. Often he tried to reason with it; and when reasoning failed, he would argue, then plead, then beg it to leave him alone, to leave him in peace. But every time Edward tried to give up, hope yanked him by the hand and told him to keep moving. If they were to get to the other side of the fire safely, they had to push on.

This morning was the first time Edward had spoken to Candy since

Levinson had given him his new T cell count in December. Maybe because the 268 put an edge of anxiety in his voice or maybe because Edward felt almost like an old friend by now, Candy passed on a new piece of intelligence. She said the AIDS unit was planning a new protease inhibitor trial; it would probably start in the spring.

Candy also said the new trial would employ a new strategy. The first Bellevue protease inhibitor study had gotten a spectacular result using indinavir alone—on average, subjects' T cell counts rose by 100 points in the study. But increasingly, researchers were beginning to think that the cancer-treatment model—using two, three, four drugs simultaneously—might also work in AIDS. The new Bellevue study would employ three drugs against HIV: the protease inhibitor, plus two other agents, AZT and 3TC. Candy said if the study came off, it would be the first time a combination therapy had been used against HIV.

"You're going to save a place for me, aren't you?" Edward asked.

"You should be a happy boy," Candy told him. "Everyone wants to get into this study and your name is first on the list."

But Edward hung up unhappy. In AIDS trials, treatment history is an important admission criterion. Nobody wants to test a new drug against a strain of virus that has already beaten other drugs. It is like beginning your boxing career by fighting the heavyweight champion. Generally, patients with limited drug exposure are preferred in trials, because they are less likely to have developed drug-resistant strains of HIV.

Candy had said a history of AZT use would be permitted in the combination study. But she did not say anything about ddI. It was possible that she simply had forgotten to mention the drug. But Edward, who had been in two studies already, thought that unlikely. Trial staff were usually very precise about admission criteria; if ddI was allowed along with AZT, Candy would have said so.

Trial staff were also very tough about enforcing admission criteria. If you had taken an "exclusion" drug, you were out of the trial, even if the alternative to being out of the trial was being dead.

.　　.　　.

A few days after the conversation with Candy, Edward had a new scare. He was driving up to Fort Lauderdale on I-95 when a slow-moving Cadillac Seville pulled into his lane from an entrance ramp. As Edward started to brake, his mind suddenly clicked out of focus. It clicked back in as the Seville was lurching into the next lane. If the other driver had not swerved when she did, Edward would have rear-ended her. "Wake up, asshole," she screamed as he passed her.

Below a 200 T cell count, Edward knew, HIV can begin to affect cognition and other brain functions. He also knew what the most common end point of brain deterioration was—AIDS-related dementia; the victim develops a wide-eyed blank stare, a slackened jaw, and an open, drooling mouth. That's how Jack Scarf had looked when Edward and Corky had brought him home to Oklahoma to die.

"My best hope now is a new drug, something the virus hasn't seen before," Edward told Sanford Levinson when he flew up to New York in mid-January.

Levinson said he agreed in principle. But there were limits to how much punishment the human body could take. "You've been in two studies already," he told Edward, "and both involved pretty toxic drugs."

Edward said he was acutely aware of his medical history. AZT, the first test drug he took, had given him stomach cramps for a year. And ddI, the experimental drug he was on now, had pushed his kidney and liver readings almost off the chart. A new drug would, very likely, bring new discomforts and dangers. But Edward was resigned to that. Over the years, he had come to think of side effects as a kind of offering you had to make periodically to the gods of HIV. It was the price you paid for staying alive.

"I need something new," Edward said. His body was already AZT resistant, and judging from his new T cell count, it was about to become ddI resistant, too. Staying alive urgently required a new drug with a new bag of tricks to throw at the virus.

Four new protease inhibitor studies were beginning in the spring, he told Levinson. Three already had a definite start date. Rockefeller University would begin a trial in May, the State University of New York in June, Columbia-Presbyterian in March. Edward said the fourth trial, the one at Bellevue, did not have an official start date, but that trial was his first choice since it would test a new strategy against the virus: a combination therapy.

Levinson said he liked the Bellevue study, too. "It's the most imaginative of the four. The combo thing just might work. What are your chances of getting in?"

"Good," Edward said. "My name is first on the candidate list. But I think ddI usage is a disqualifier." Edward paused and raised an eyebrow. "I believe that was your idea, the ddI trial."

Levinson ignored the remark. "Who told you ddI was a disqualification?"

Edward mentioned the conversation with Candy.

"Ah, but she didn't say ddI would rule you out. Why don't you ask her?"

The question struck Edward as astonishingly stupid. "*Sandy*, if I tell Candy I'm on ddI, and it is a disqualifier, I'm out on my ass. You know that."

"Edward, what if you tell her that you're just curious. You just want to know if ddI use is a trial exclusion."

"Then Candy becomes suspicious. She wonders why I'm asking about ddI. She tells her boss, and I'm out. Do you know how many people want to get into this study? Thousands."

Levinson looked at him for a moment. "You want to know what I'd do?"

"What?" Edward said.

"Lie, lie, lie."

CHAPTER FOUR

C. Everett Koop was stunned.

The new surgeon general had encountered exactly two cases of *Pneumocystis carinii* pneumonia in the first forty years of his career. Now, suddenly, within the space of a month, March 1981, five documented cases of PCP had come across his desk. The infection pattern was also very strange; all five cases had occurred in the same city, Los Angeles, and within the same population group, young gay men.

A few months later, Dr. Thomas Waldman, an immunologist at the National Cancer Institute, also encountered a medical rarity. An NCI clinical ward had just admitted a patient with *Candida albicans*, a rare fungal infection. There was no question about the accuracy of the diagnosis; the patient, a young man, had the classic sign of *Candida* fungal: a white frothlike substance around the mouth, throat, and fingernails. What was strange was the patient's susceptibility; the young man's immune system should have been able to destroy the fungus easily. Why hadn't it?

About the same time, Dr. David Auerbach, an investigator in the Los Angeles office of the Centers for Disease Control, encountered a bizarre statistical fluke. One day a visitor, the leader of an L.A. gay group, showed Dr. Auerbach a photo of ten smiling young men taken at a gay charity benefit two years earlier. Four of the men in the picture were dead now, the visitor said, all from the same disease, Kaposi's sarcoma. What were the odds of something like that happening? he asked.

Dr. Auerbach thought for a minute, then said there was less than a 1 percent chance that four men in their early and mid-thirties would die within a twenty-four-month period. The odds that all four would die of Kaposi's sarcoma, a rare form of cancer, were too low to be calculated.

In that same year, 1981, what was eventually to be called AIDS—Acquired Immune Deficiency Syndrome—made its debut in the medical literature; and considering its dramatic subsequent history, the debut was relatively modest. A brief piece in the June 16 issue of the Centers for Disease Control's journal, *Mortality and Morbidity Weekly Report (MMWR)*, took note of the five cases of PCP among homosexual men that had surprised Dr. Koop. A few weeks later, the July 4 issue of *MMWR* described a puzzling complex of hitherto unassociated diseases that had begun to appear among gay men in San Francisco, Los Angeles, and New York.

In part the *MMWR* article read:

> The occurrence of twenty-six cases of Kaposi's sarcoma (KS) during a thirty-month period among young homosexual men is considered highly unusual. . . . That ten new cases of *Pneumocystis carinii* pneumonia (PCP) have been identified in homosexual men suggests that the five previously reported cases were not an isolated phenomenon. . . . In addition, CDC has a report of four homosexual men in New York City who developed severe progressive perianal herpes simplex infection and had evidence of cellular immuno-deficiency. . . . It is not clear if or how the clustering of KS, *Pneumocystis* pneumonia and other serious diseases in homosexual men are related.

Almost every investigator who looked into what was being called the "gay disease" noticed one similarity. A healthy immune system could easily destroy all of the diseases that compromised it. So the "gay disease" must be an immune disorder of some type. But what could cause it?

One early suspect was amyl nitrate, a drug widely used by gay men in the early 1980s to enhance sexual pleasure. Another was anal intercourse. Some researchers thought that sperm deposited in the anus during gay sex might produce an allergic reaction that would somehow compromise the immune system.

However, a 1982 New York University conference suggested that the "gay disease" might have a non-gay cause after all. Everyone came to the NYU meeting prepared to discuss the usual suspects—sperm, amyl nitrate, the "homosexual lifestyle." But a five-minute presentation by Dr. William Folger, then head of the CDC, changed everyone's thinking. Dr. Folger announced that the next issue of *MMWR* would publish the first documented cases of the "gay disease" in a nonhomosexual population, hemophiliacs; the hemophiliacs had been infected via blood transfusion, Dr. Folger said. This was precisely the news the medical community had been dreading. It meant that the "gay disease" was probably caused by a viral agent, and since the disease was new, the virus was likely new, too. Worst of all, the outbreak among hemophiliacs—frequent recipients of blood transfusions—indicated that the mysterious virus was now in the nation's blood supply.

According to Randy Shilts in *And the Band Played On*, Dr. Don Francis, another CDC official, was the first American scientist to suspect that a retrovirus might be responsible for AIDS. Most living things replicate by transforming DNA, the genetic code of life, into RNA, and then into proteins. Retroviruses, which were originally thought to occur only in animals, reverse the process (hence, the name retro). They carry their genetic code in the form of RNA.

Dr. Francis noticed an intriguing parallel between AIDS and feline leukemia, an animal retroviral disease. Both diseases created an unusual vulnerability to secondary infection. In animals, as in humans, T4 (or helper T) cells function like the quarterback of the immune system: T4 cells coordinate the system's response to infectious agents. Secondary infections occur frequently in feline leukemia because the feline retro-virus kills T cells, leaving the cat vulnerable to invasion by usually easy-to-destroy viruses and microbes. Did AIDS victims fall prey to PCP, cytomegalovirus (CMV), and other secondary infections for the same reason? Was a retrovirus also killing their T cells?

In 1981, only one human retrovirus, HTLV (human T cell lym-photropic virus), had been identified, so it immediately came under suspicion. But Dr. Robert Gallo, discoverer of HTLV and director of research at the National Cancer Institute, came up with a paradoxical finding when he began to look for HTLV in AIDS patients: blood sam-ples of patients with the "gay disease" showed evidence of retroviral in-fection, but Dr. Gallo could not find any actual virus in the samples. A second NCI study only deepened the mystery. HTLV is character-ized by massive, out-of-control T4 cell production, but AIDS patients seemed to have the opposite problem; the blood samples Dr. Gallo examined contained barely any T cells at all.

There is still some dispute about who identified HIV first—a French team led by Dr. Luc Montagnier of the Pasteur Institute in Paris, or Dr. Gallo in a later wave of studies—but by the end of 1983, a little more than eighteen months after the outbreak of the HIV epidemic, the virus had been identified and given a name: Human Immunodeficiency Virus.

In 1984, it became clear that HIV was not a high-contagion agent. It could not be spread by personal contact, i.e., through kissing, or via toilet seats or other kinds of routine daily contact, but only through blood, se-men, or needle exchange. In a feat of epidemiological wizardry, re-searchers also identified the person who may have ignited the AIDS outbreak. In the charts of government epidemiologists (doctors who study disease trends and patterns), he is identified as Patient Zero. His real name is Gaetan Dugas, and in *And the Band Played On*, Randy Shilts describes him as a promiscuous, heartbreakingly handsome, sandy-haired French Canadian with a profession ideally suited to spreading a new virus. Dugas, an airline steward for Air Canada, was a regular visitor to New York, San Francisco, and Los Angeles. Of the first 106 men diagnosed with AIDS in the United States, forty-two had had sex with Dugas.

In 1984, AIDS's most disturbing characteristic was also becoming increasingly clear: No one survived it. Half of the 12,000 Americans diagnosed as HIV positive since the epidemic's outbreak were dead by 1985. A decade later, the death toll stood at 320,000 and the HIV-infection rate at almost a million. AIDS, the second leading cause of death among Americans between the ages of twenty-five and forty-four, had by the mid-1990s begun to reach plaguelike proportions in some communities. In 1996, HIV accounted for 40 percent of deaths among African-American men, and 20 percent among African-American women, between the ages twenty-five and forty-four.

Most experts believe that HIV, like the Marburg and Ebola viruses, originated in Central Africa, where it was common in certain species of primates. According to this theory, the first animal-man transfer took place about a century ago and may have occurred when a hunter became infected by the blood of a dead or dying animal. Mathematical models suggest that, up until the second half of the twentieth century, the virus spread very slowly, but two changes suddenly gave it "legs." The first was the creation of a worldwide airline network. The virus could now hop on a plane and be anywhere on earth within twenty-four hours. In a recent paper delivered at a conference on AIDS at the National Institutes of Health, Dr. Bernardino Fantini, a professor of history and medicine at the University of Rome, described the second change this way.

I would argue that during the second half of the twentieth century, the effective transmission of the virulent AIDS virus has been favored by the introduction of new ways of diffusion, such as blood transfusion, wider use of injected drugs, sexual promiscuity, and thanks to new medical breakthroughs, the increasing survival of infected people. This association of biological and social factors has caused a breach in the wall, which in the past protected the human race against the catastrophic spread of infectious diseases.

No one has ever fully succeeded in articulating the awful physical agony of AIDS, but in *Angels in America*, playwright Tony Kushner comes close. One of his characters, consumed by the disease, describes his suffering in the following way:

> God splits the skin with a jagged thumbnail from throat to belly and then plunges a huge filthy hand in. He grabs hold of your body tubes, and they slip to evade his grasp. But he squeezes hard, he insists. He pulls and pulls until all of your innards are yanked out, and then he stuffs them back in, dirty, tangled, torn. It's up to you to do the stitching.

Generally, the initial HIV infection precedes the onset of symptoms by five to eight years. Like a spacecraft locking onto a mother ship, free-floating HIV locks onto the CD4 receptor site of a passing helper T cell. Other types of cells also possess receptor sites, but nature, through some design fluke, has created a perfect lock-and-key fit between the T cells and HIV. Without the cell's genetic machinery, HIV cannot replicate, so the virus inserts its genes inside the core of the T cell. To penetrate the cell membrane, the virus first transforms its RNA-based genetic code into the more universal DNA-based code. This is accomplished via an enzyme called reverse transcriptase, which the virus carries with it. The new retroviral DNA then acts the way the pod people did in 1950s science fiction movies. HIV migrates to the nucleus of the T cell, where it inserts its DNA into the T cell's DNA.

True infection occurs when the T cell, following the more universal replication process, begins to convert its DNA into long, thin strands of RNA. In a healthy T4 cell, the RNA then encodes for proteins, which the old cell uses to construct a new cell. In an infected cell, the new proteins become building blocks of HIV. Sometimes the virus will remain dormant for years inside a cell; other times the newly minted HIV will migrate to the T cell's outer wall, bud off, and begin to search for other T cells to infect. Typically, the old infected cell will then explode and die.

A small group of HIV-positive individuals remains healthy fifteen to twenty years after infection, but they are the exception; usually HIV works more quickly. As basketball star Magic Johnson did, almost half of HIV-positive men and women suffer flulike symptoms in the first two to twelve weeks after infection. The fever, chills, and tiredness that characterize an HIV flu are signs of an aroused immune system, which often will kill 90 to 95 percent of HIV during its first attack. But the surviving 5 to 10 percent continues to wage a guerrilla action—usually from the body's lymph system; at first the action is low level, but as HIV replenishes itself, the action intensifies until finally, full-scale war breaks out. According to Dr. Anthony Fauci, director of AIDS research at the National Institute of Allergies and Infectious Diseases, one year postinfection, the typical patient's T cell count is 600 T cells per microliter of blood. Three years postinfection, it is 400 to 500, and seven years postinfection—roughly where Edward was in the late winter of 1995 before the start of the Bellevue trial—the individual's count is often in the high 200s.

The reason 200 is considered the official dividing line between HIV infection and HIV disease is that below a 200 T cell count the immune system becomes too weak to mount a defense against normally easy-to-kill opportunistic infections; 200 is the point at which the fire begins.

As at the epidemic's beginning, *Pneumocystis carinii* pneumonia (PCP) remains a leading form of opportunistic infection and also a leading cause of death in AIDS, though, thanks to new treatments (and the use of prophylactic therapy), this secondary invader isn't nearly as lethal as it used to be. In the early and mid-1980s, 80 percent of AIDS patients experienced at least one episode of PCP, and the majority never recovered from it. Today, the infection is a factor in less than 20 percent of deaths. So vulnerable is the PCP microbe to T cell attack that, even at the 300 level, the body is usually able to contain it. But once T cells fall into the 200 range, the microbe is free to set up shop in the heart, kidneys, and its favorite site, the lungs. There it lodges in the air sacs used by the body to transfer oxygen from inhaled breath into the bloodstream. As these tiny airholes are clogged by a thin layer of white mucus, the individual starts to feel as if he were breathing though a thick wool blanket. As more and more sacs block up, breathing becomes progressively harder; the individual feels as if he were trying to draw breath through two, four, eight, and then, finally, a dozen thick wool blankets.

Cytomegalovirus (CMV), another leading form of opportunistic infection, can also cause pneumonia, as well as ravage the nervous system and gastrointestinal tract. But like PCP, CMV has favorite targets; one is the retina of the eye. At about the 50 to 100 T cell level, the world suddenly begins to grow darker for about 20 percent of AIDS patients. The dimming effect, the first sign of CMV retinitis, is caused by leatherlike gray lesions on the peripheral regions of the retina. The lesions are created by clumps of dead cells killed by CMV and by the leakage of protein. As the virus penetrates farther into the retina, lesions appear in the macular portion of the optic disc. At this point, dimness begins to turn to darkness; the victim feels as if he were wearing sunglasses all the time. Total blindness, often an end point of CMV retinitis, usually develops when the hard little knots of dead cells in the optic disc thicken to a cataractlike density.

The toxoplasmosis parasite is another threat to patients with low T cell counts. Carried in cats, toxoplasmosis parasites attack the heart, lungs, and spleen. However, the favorite target of the parasite is the brain. One of the saddest sights in AIDS hospices are twenty-five- and thirty-year-olds who suddenly find the simple acts of daily life incredibly strenuous. Someone with a toxoplasmosis-ravaged brain may need as long as thirty seconds to summon up the mental concentration to pick up a fork from the table. As the disease progresses, behaviors become progressively disjointed and discrete. Now after picking up the fork, the individual has to pause again and remuster his concentration for the next act: putting the fork into the food. In the later stages of central-nervous-system toxoplasmosis, a simple activity like getting out of bed and getting dressed becomes a jumble of a hundred separate behaviors that can take up to an hour to perform. Typically, brain scans done at this stage of the disease show that the toxoplasmosis parasite has already eaten away 10 percent to 15 percent of the brain mass.

Dementia, another neurological disorder common in AIDS, is caused, at least in part, by HIV itself. Seemingly innocent memory lapses are its calling card, but as the dementia progresses, the victim becomes subject to headaches and violent, epileptic-like seizures. Unlike toxoplasmosis, dementia sometimes destroys the "I" that defines selfhood. In late-stage dementia, the face and body often come to look uninhabited. The eyes are vacant, the mouth open and expressionless, the arms and legs slack and energyless. Seeing a seventy-year-old in this state is heartrending; seeing a twenty-two-year-old like this calls into question the notion of a merciful God.

Kaposi's sarcoma, named after its discoverer, Moritz Kaposi, a nineteenth-century Viennese medical luminary, typically appears on the limbs first, as clusters of reddish-brown nodules. In his original report on KS, Kaposi noted that the disease's outward progression is mirrored internally; nodules also begin to appear in "the lung, liver, heart, spleen, and gastrointestinal tract, producing fever, bloody diarrhea, and coughing of blood . . . followed by death." Until the emergence of HIV, KS, which is caused by a member of the herpes family of viruses, used to be relatively rare; the medical literature of the nineteenth century contains only a hundred cases; and all of them were among Mediterranean men—Italians, Greeks, and Jews—of an advanced age.

Today, KS is a multicultural disease and its victims tend to be under forty-five years old.

Besides lethality, most of the diseases associated with AIDS share one other characteristic: They kill the human body in terrible ways. With HIV, there is almost no such thing as a good death.

CHAPTER FIVE

AFTER YEARS OF DISAPPOINTMENT AND DESPAIR, YEARS OF FRUSTRA-
tion and impotence, in January 1995 hope was in the brisk winter air.
Finally, a new therapy was on the horizon that could tame AIDS, could
bring it under control, could transform it from a killer into a manageable chronic disease like diabetes or hypertension.

Maybe.

The first generation of AIDS drugs: AZT, ddI, ddC—all the agents
developed in the late eighties and early nineties—possessed a singular
drawback. They all attacked the virus at the same point in its replication cycle. And since some HIV always survived the attack, the drugs
could produce only temporary remissions. The residue of resistant
virus in the body would quickly reproduce, and six months, nine
months, a year later, the cycle of suffering and morbidity would begin
all over again.

In early 1994, word began to spread through the medical and HIV
communities about a new drug with a new plan of attack. In December
of that year, a National Institutes of Health official, Dr. Margaret John-

son, told the *Wall Street Journal* that protease inhibitors represented the most exciting new development in AIDS treatment in the past decade.

The Bellevue trial, Edward's trial, would be among the first to pair indinavir, one of the most promising of the new inhibitors, with other drugs: AZT, a veteran anti-AIDS agent, and 3TC, a newer chemical cousin of AZT. In the Bellevue trial, AZT and 3TC would block reverse transcriptase, the enzyme HIV needs for the first step in its replication process: the transformation of its RNA into DNA. However, the real star of the study would be indinavir (trade name Crixivan), which would, in theory at least, kill the strains of virus that outwitted AZT and 3TC.

In drug company promotional literature, pharmaceutical research is depicted as a high-tech marvel. But during the first desperate years of the AIDS epidemic, most companies were reduced to the most primitive trial-and-error research methods. Essentially, researchers just put the virus in a petri dish, then, one by one, put every drug in the company's inventory into the dish and hoped something would happen. Occasionally, the method turned up an agent of value; the HIV-fighting properties of AZT, originally an anticancer drug, were discovered via the hit-and-miss method. But more often—much more often—the method only wasted valuable time.

Instead of randomly throwing existing drugs at the virus, in 1986, Irving Sigal, Merck's director of biomedical research, decided to reverse the process. He believed that the quickest route to an effective AIDS therapy would be to identify HIV's genetic weak points, then design a specific class of drugs to attack them. But did the seemingly invincible virus possess any weaknesses? The genetic map Sigal and his team produced in 1987—the first ever of HIV's internal structure—showed that the virus did indeed; and two points appeared to be particularly vulnerable to drug intervention.

However, the first point, located early in the HIV replication cycle, was already under attack. AZT, ddI, and all the other early anti-AIDS agents, were designed to block reverse transcriptase, the enzyme HIV needs to convert its RNA into DNA.

The other major weak point in the replication cycle was near the end. The virus emerges from the T cell's DNA nucleus looking like a pearl necklace laid out lengthwise on a table. In order to mature— which is to say, in order to infect other T cells—the pearls, which are really individual proteins, have to be cut apart. Another HIV enzyme, protease, does the cutting. Protease acts as a kind of chemical scissors. Inhibit the production of protease and the virus won't die, but the proteins will remain uncut, immature, and harmless.

In 1987, other drug companies were also trying to develop agents that could inhibit protease production. But there was a great opportunity for an aggressive research team, particularly one with a knack for genetic mapping.

In the late 1980s, a lobster-claw structure began to appear on computer screens in Merck labs. The claw, the first three-dimensional picture of an HIV protease, indicated that the enzyme had two vulnerabilities. The claw was made from two separate structures; prevent the two structures from fusing together and there would be no claw and thus no way for the virus to cut the HIV proteins on the necklace. The second vulnerable site was inside the claw. Prevent its jaws from snapping shut and you produce the same result. No cleaving action, no mature HIV, and hence, no AIDS.

Merck's mapmaking skills gave it a sizable early lead in the race to develop a protease inhibitor. But then Irving Sigal was killed. The thirty-five-year-old scientist was a passenger on Pan Am flight 103, which was blown up by a terrorist bomb over Lockerbee, Scotland, in December 1988. In 1993, the indinavir development program suffered a second setback; the drug turned in a surprisingly disappointing performance in one of its first human trials, trial 006, a relatively small study of HIV-positive subjects.

At the start of the trial, Emilio Emini, director of antiviral research at Merck and a driving force on the indinavir project, was very optimistic. Laboratory studies indicated that Merck's new designer drug could do everything an effective protease inhibitor needed to do. In the test tube, it inhibited the binding process that fused the two sides of the enzyme into a lobster claw, and in cases in which the two sides did manage to fuse, it inhibited their ability to open and close in a scissorlike motion. Early lab data also suggested that Merck chemists might have solved the problem that, to varying degrees, had undermined the effectiveness of every other AIDS drug—viral resistance.

One paradoxical quality of HIV is its profound stupidity. Most viruses make one or two mistakes during replication, but dim-witted HIV routinely makes dozens. It forgets to add a protein here, puts in an extra enzyme over there; it is constantly confused, constantly screwing up, and as a result, constantly producing mutant strains of itself. If our genes were as stupid as HIV's, people with six heads, eight toes, and four feet would be common. But in an ironic twist on Darwinian theory, HIV's single-digit IQ turns out to be a very effective adaptive mechanism. The reason? The high mutation rate of the virus gives it an almost infinite capacity for reinvention. Every time a drug threatens to kill it, HIV quickly morphs into a new, unkillable form. AZT, ddI— every agent thrown against the virus has followed the same course. Each works for a while; then a mutant viral strain emerges, and the drug begins to lose effectiveness.

Emini's hopes that indinavir would be different were based on its lab performance. In a petri dish, HIV seemed incapable of mutating strains that could stand up to the drug. However, early returns from trial 006 showed that the virus was more agile in the human body. As with most other anti-AIDS agents, at first indinavir wreaked havoc, but after a four-to-six-month interval, its effectiveness began to wane. Apparently, the virus's stupidity had saved it again.

The early data from 006 did contain one encouraging result. Along with drug resistance, the subjects' immune systems appeared to grow healthier as the study progressed. This paradox suggested that there might be a simple reason for the resistance problem: not enough indinavir. Emini and his team doubled the trial dose to 2,400 mg per day. That worked. At the 2.4 mg level—given from day one of therapy—indinavir produced a large drop in viral load (the amount of active virus in the blood) and a substantial increase in T cell count, and sustained both changes over the remaining eight months of the study. The viral resistance problem continued, but trial 006's final results showed that the problem had been substantially mitigated.

Despite the good news, no one at Merck believed that a protease inhibitor alone could tame AIDS, turn it from a sure killer into a manageable chronic disease. Experience showed that even the most potent and promising new drugs perform best as part of a team, as part of a one-two punch therapy. But what drugs would make the best allies for indinavir?

In October 1994, Schlomo Staszewski, a leading German researcher, leaned across the table of a crowded Frankfurt restaurant and asked his luncheon companion if he planned to attend the International AIDS Conference in Glasgow the following month. When Ferdinand Massari, director of clinical research at Merck, said no, Staszewski told him he should. One of the papers being given at the conference would interest him; it was on 3TC, a new anti-AIDS agent.

Massari was intrigued. A lead researcher in the first European trials of 3TC, Staszewski knew a lot about the drug. The German also knew that in its first combination trial, indinavir had been let down badly by its two partners; AZT and ddI had produced so much GI distress—a familiar side effect of both drugs—that many subjects had dropped out of the trial.

Could Staszewski be hinting that 3TC would make a better partner for indinavir?

In October 1994, all Massari knew about 3TC was that it was a new-generation reverse-transcriptase inhibitor, and supposedly much easier to tolerate than AZT and ddI. A scheduling conflict made it impossible for him to go to Glasgow himself, but Massari thought someone from Merck should be at the conference. On his return to the company's research headquarters in Pennsylvania, he spoke to John Ryan, head of the clinical trials department. A few days later, Jeff Chodakewitz, a young Merck scientist, was given the Glasgow assignment.

The meeting confirmed the rumors about 3TC's safety. According to one conference report, 3TC and its partner AZT produced almost no side effects, a remarkable accomplishment in an area of medicine where drug tolerance was a serious problem. Preliminary data also indicated that 3TC was more effective against HIV than the existing reverse-transcriptase inhibitors. More unexpectedly, in the European trials, 3TC seemed to have a supercharger effect on AZT. Normally, as the virus develops resistance, AZT's effectiveness wanes. But the combination of 3TC and AZT kept AZT active longer.

As he sat in the audience at Glasgow, Chodakewitz recalled a conversation he and Massari had had before he left for Scotland. The two men had found themselves speculating about whether science had, quite serendipitously, already assembled all the tools necessary to tame AIDS. Back in Pennsylvania, that possibility had seemed like idle office chatter, but here in Glasgow, it suddenly began to seem real. The capacity of AZT and 3TC to deliver a powerful first punch (inhibit production of reverse transcriptase) combined with indinavir's ability to deliver a powerful second punch (inhibit the protease enzyme's ability to cleave) might make it possible to transform AIDS from a progressive terminal illness into a manageable chronic condition like hypertension or diabetes.

After Chodakewitz's return from the conference, an idea that had been floating around Merck for several months—pairing up indinavir with 3TC and AZT in a clinical trial—suddenly took on new urgency. On December 23, 1994—five days before Edward received his new T cell count—Dr. Chodakewitz's proposal for a clinical trial of the three agents was green-lighted by Merck. Four days later, the study received an official number, 035, and a starting date: late spring or early summer 1995. In the world of medical clinical trials, this was the equivalent of moving at the speed of light.

Immediately after the new year, Chodakewitz drew up a design for 035. Trials that employ a placebo and are double-blind (i.e., neither the investigators nor the subjects know who is getting what) generally produce the most scientifically reliable results. But because of the ethical concerns in AIDS trials, Merck, like most pharmaceutical companies, does not use placebos. Chodakewitz's design ensured that everyone would get something. One-third of the 035 subjects would receive the true therapy, the 3TC-AZT-indinavir combination; one-third the protease inhibitor alone (plus two bottles of placebos, one marked AZT, one 3TC); and one-third the 3TC-AZT combination (plus a bottle of placebos marked indinavir).

Next, Chodakewitz had to make a decision about trial candidates. "Therapy-naive individuals" (i.e., untreated individuals) would make the best subjects. The three-drug combination might produce dramatic results in subjects who had not developed AZT-resistant strains of HIV. But the organized AIDS community—a force to be reckoned with in all decisions about HIV therapy—might object to such a narrow selection criteria. And even if the community did not object, were there enough untreated HIV-positive individuals in the United States in 1995 to fill up a study? At the very least, finding untreated men and women would be a recruitment nightmare. Chodakewitz decided to make pregnancy, a history of alcohol or drug abuse, a hepatitis B infection, or a T cell count above 400 or below 50 exclusions. Everything Edward was worried about and determined to hide—including ddI use—was in fact permitted.

No one had ever taken AZT, 3TC, and indinavir in combination before, and while side effects were not expected to be a major problem, expecting was not the same as knowing. Death is a rare but not unknown side effect in research medicine. As a safety precaution, Chodakewitz decided that a pretrial safety test should precede 035 proper. In late spring or earlier if possible, the first twenty-four of 035's ninety subjects would begin taking the combination therapy. If no one died or sustained serious injury, 035 proper would start eight weeks later. As a further safety precaution, an elaborate set of screening and monitoring procedures was established. Trial candidates would be required to take three different types of physical exams (including an extensive ophthalmological exam) and submit to fifteen different kinds of lab tests. For the first three months, subjects' T cell counts and viral assays (tests that measure the amount of active virus in the blood) would be taken weekly; for the next three months, biweekly; for the remainder of the year-long trial, monthly. Everyone, including participants, would have access to T cell data, but the results of the viral-load assays, which measure the amount of active HIV in the blood, would be blind; only Merck scientists would have access to them while the trial was running.

Chodakewitz's next decision, the trial's size, was complicated by a phenomenon almost unique to AIDS clinical trials: cheating. No one knows how frequently people cheat to get into AIDS studies, but Chodakewitz thinks that it may happen more frequently among AIDS patients because they are more medically sophisticated than most patients and more aggressive in searching out new treatments. Ferdinand Massari believes the cheating problem has deeper roots: "The gay community's history as a marginalized and sometimes persecuted minority has encouraged a distrust of authority," Massari says. "So often, HIV subjects are less willing to follow instructions than other types of patients."

Chodakewitz decided that ninety patients, fifteen to twenty more than he needed, would provide him with an adequate margin to overcome the faulty data any cheating might produce.

In mid-January, the University of North Carolina Medical Center, the University of Pittsburgh, the University of California at San Diego, and Bellevue were chosen as the four 035 test sites. At the first three sites, experienced investigators would head the trial units. But Roy (Trip) Gulick, the young researcher who was deputy director of the AIDS clinical trials unit at Bellevue had never run a major study before.

Normally, Chodakewitz would have hesitated before appointing an inexperienced young researcher as a principal investigator (PI) at a test site. But during 006, Gulick had impressed him. He had a good eye for detail, was conscientious and methodical, and reported problems quickly—something not all clinical investigators do. Furthermore, when Charles Farthing, head of the Bellevue unit, left for UCLA midway through 006, Gulick had stepped in and navigated the study to a successful conclusion.

On January 15, Chodakewitz called Gulick and offered him the PI spot at Bellevue. The two men talked for a while, then Chodakewitz said half jokingly that if Bellevue got the trial up and running before the other three sites, he would make Gulick PI for the entire study. Gulick decided to ignore the jokey tone of the offer.

"I can launch by April twenty-eighth," he said.

"That's only three months away, Trip."

"I can do it."

"Well, Speedy Gonzales, you do it and you get to be PI for the whole study."

Chodakewitz's tone was still playful. Nonetheless, the PI position on a major trial like 035 would be a real prize, a real career maker. Studies like 035—if they succeeded—could turn you into a marquee name overnight.

Everyone—newspapers, television, and newsweeklies—would want to talk to the head of a breakthrough AIDS trial.

"April twenty-eighth, Jeff," Gulick said again, then hung up.

CHAPTER SIX

"MY NAME IS JO—" THE YOUNG MAN WAS TOO OUT OF BREATH TO FIN-
ish the sentence. He opened his mouth and heaved his chest upward;
suddenly, a horrible sucking sound filled the emergency room. The
young man tried to breathe again; he wheezed, he rocked back and
forth, but nothing worked; oxygen refused to pass through his lips into
his lungs. Bewildered, he looked at the nurse, a large, motherly black
woman, then at the slim young doctor standing beside her. Suddenly,
the young man's head snapped back again. More horrible sucking
sounds. Then his frail body began to shake; it had reached the limits of
its endurance. The young man collapsed, in slow motion, backward
onto the ER gurney.

Two ER workers removed his sweat-soaked shirt; then the nurse
placed an oxygen mask over his face. It slipped; the young man's skin
was too wet. The nurse toweled his face dry and tried again. This time
the mask stayed.

Resident Trip Gulick had worked in the ER for ten months. But
this was the first time he had seen someone his own age dying. The

artificially administered oxygen would buy a little extra time, but within twelve to eighteen hours, the gray-white blanket of PCP mucus in the young man's lungs would become impenetrable. He was going to die, to suffocate in a bubbly field of his own mucus and there was nothing anyone could do to save him. As Dr. Gulick watched an orderly wheel the young man out of the ER, he thought how alike the two of them were— he and the gasping, desperate, bewildered figure on the gurney. Two educated young gay men separated by nothing more than a stroke of fate.

Dr. Gulick is not a big believer in life-transforming epiphanies. But as he watched the young man's gurney disappear into the crowded hospital corridor, he knew how he would spend the rest of his medical career.

In an odd way, the two—the disease and the doctor—have had parallel careers. In 1982, nine months after the first cases of PCP were reported, Dr. Gulick graduated from Columbia University's College of Physicians and Surgeons, and in 1986, the year the virus killed its twenty-five thousandth American, he was made Harvard Medical School's first postdoctoral fellow in AIDS. Nineteen eighty-six was also a memorable year for another reason; before leaving for Boston that summer, Dr. Gulick told his father, a retired Marine Corps colonel, that he was gay.

In the early 1990s, Dr. Gulick decided that he could make a larger contribution to the fight against AIDS as an investigator than as a private physician. This decision led him first to Beth Israel Hospital in Boston, where he worked as a junior researcher, then to New York University Medical Center, where he was appointed deputy director of the Bellevue AIDS Clinical Trials Unit in 1992. If the war against AIDS has a front line, it runs through big city municipal hospitals like Bellevue and San Francisco General. But even at Bellevue, the front of the front lines, the life of a junior officer consists of unglamorous drudge work; during his first years at the AIDS trials unit, Dr. Gulick monitored subjects, filled out forms, answered questions . . .

Jeff Chodakewitz's call could change all that.

But to win the title of principal investigator on trial 035, Dr. Gulick would have to perform a small miracle of organization. A study normally takes twelve to eighteen months to organize and launch. He had barely three months to have the safety study for 035 up and operating. Recruitment would not be a problem. Candy Talcbucon's phone log already contained hundreds of names, and once word of 035 leaked out, the trials unit would be inundated with calls. But forty or fifty people would have to be screened to find twelve suitable candidates for the safety study, the first portion of the trial, and maybe another 200 to fill the fifteen other spots Bellevue had available when trial 035 proper began eight weeks later. An announcement of the trial should be made now.

But in mid-January, two weeks after he had spoken to Chodakewitz, all Dr. Gulick had in hand was a rough draft of the trial protocol (a list of 035's rules and regulations); announcing the study now was risky. The company could still cancel the trial before the official draft of the protocol was issued in early February. At Beth Israel in Boston, Dr. Gulick had seen what the last-minute cancellation of a study could do to AIDS patients. Three extra weeks of recruiting and screening time would have been useful. But the researcher decided that losing the time—and maybe the PI title—was better than making another round of calls like the ones he had had to make in Boston.

However, the AIDS grapevine was already way ahead of him. The week of January 20, the trials unit received a dozen inquiries about the study. The week after that, several dozen. The week that 035 was officially announced—the week of February 2—Candy logged 150 calls, the week after that 200. On February 23, when she stopped counting, approximately 400 people had made inquiries about the twenty-seven available spots. Some callers had friends in high places. A high-level White House official contacted Dr. Gulick's boss, Dr. Fred Valentine, on behalf of one applicant.

Candy would tell out-of-state and out-of-country callers that weekly visits to Bellevue would be required for the first three months of the trial, but no one seemed to mind. Callers said they were willing to fly into New York once a week or even to move there.

On February 17, Dr. Gulick made a controversial decision. Geographical proximity would make adverse reactions easier to monitor and treat. So he decided to limit participation in trial 035 to metropolitan New York residents.

One hundred applicants, including Edward, survived the residency cut, but there were still nearly four people for every trial spot—each more desperate than the next, and each more certain than the next that trial 035 represented his last, best hope. Competition for the twenty-seven trial spots would be determined by the following criteria: a T cell count of between 50 and 400, a viral load of under 20,000 (i.e., 20,000 copies of HIV per millimeter of blood), no previous episodes of full-blown AIDS, no serious preexisting illnesses such as heart disease, cancer, diabetes, hepatitis, or retinitis, and no previous experience with a protease inhibitor or 3TC.

At the end of February, an informed-consent form was given to the candidates who came closest to fulfilling these criteria; it outlined the objectives of trial 035 and listed the potential dangers of the three test drugs.

A note on page two explained that nine patients would be randomly assigned the indinavir-AZT-3TC combination that was potentially the most effective therapy: nine to the protease inhibitor combination; and nine to the AZT and 3TC combination. No one—including Dr. Gulick—would know who was getting what until trial 035 ended.

The form also described the potential side effects of each test drug. Indinavir's included diarrhea, vomiting, fatigue, dizziness, jaundice, hematuria (blood in the urine), and renal colic (pain in the kidneys). But since protease inhibitors were a new class of drug, participants were warned that this list of adverse reactions could grow.

Headaches, muscle aches, nausea, vomiting, diarrhea, rash, fever, and a decreased white and red blood cell count were listed as AZT's principal side effects. But the consent form also made a cryptic reference to "other," less common side effects associated with the drug.

The principal side effects of 3TC were headache, diarrhea, fatigue, nausea, insomnia, fever, abdominal pain, rash, and a decreased red and white blood cell count.

Page three of the form noted that final acceptance into the study was contingent on an overall general exam, an EKG (to measure cardiac function), a chest X ray, and an ophthalmological checkup (primarily to check for the presence of CMV retinitis). T cell counts and viral loads would be monitored during the general physical and then again when subjects came in for the EKG and chest X ray. Complete blood counts and blood chemistries also would be taken during these visits. The twelve subjects selected for the safety study would have to undergo one additional screening procedure—a day of hour-by-hour monitoring.

When Edward received his consent form at the end of February, he immediately flipped to page four and ran his finger down the list of exclusions. Pregnancy . . . hepatitis . . . alcohol abuse . . . immuno-suppressive therapy . . . ddI was not on the list. Maybe he was being paranoid. Maybe the drug was not an exclusion after all. On the other hand, the form did say "Use of any investigational agent is an exclusionary factor." Conceivably, that phrase could apply to ddI.

Edward took a sip of his coffee and looked across Ocean Drive. The beach was filling up early this morning.

Should he call Candy? He took another sip of coffee. No, he decided, too risky. Questions about ddI might make her suspicious. Better to stick with the plan he and Levinson had worked out on the phone the other night: Don't mention the Columbia-Presbyterian study and stop taking ddI now so the last traces of the drug would be out of his system when he flew up to New York on March 29 for his first screening appointment.

Edward felt guilty about the plan. Researchers were always complaining about how cheating compromised test results. But he was fighting for his life, wasn't he? It was easy to be high-minded when you had a 1,400 T cell count. But he didn't; he was in a war. And when you were in a war, only one thing mattered: winning.

"Never mind the goddamn study, Edward, your first responsibility is to yourself," Levinson had told him the other night on the phone. Levinson could be a pain in the ass, but he was gay. And you could trust a gay doctor. They knew whose side they were on.

Edward picked up the consent form again and read the attached note. Apparently, the principal investigator, Dr. Roy Gulick, wanted to see some proof of his New York State residency. The calls from down here were already arousing suspicions about his legal residence. Why rouse them further with questions about ddI? Levinson was right: Don't volunteer any information and, if necessary, "lie, lie, lie."

Edward picked up *The New York Times* from the coffee table, creased it carefully down the middle, and opened it. Edward read newspapers the way he did everything else: methodically. News stories, the business section, and arts first, then the society pages (on Sunday), and finally, what recently had become an extension of the society pages for Edward, the obituaries. It amused him to see who came out in death and who did not. Over the years, he had noticed two distinct trends. The most open of the famous and nearly famous would list AIDS as the cause of death and, if there was one, a lover as next of kin; the least candid, a parent as next of kin and an unrelated illness as the cause of death. In the early and mid-eighties, Edward had noticed a sudden rash of brain tumors and pneumonia among men in their thirties, forties, and early fifties.

Edward was still uncertain what he would do about his own obituary. In 1989, in a fit of spite, he had torn up the notice his former employer, the European petroleum company, had prepared for him. But recently, Edward had begun to have second thoughts. He had no close family, no children, no longtime lover to bear witness to his life. Did he really want to go without leaving at least one tiny fingerprint behind, one small notice that Edward Sandisfield had spent some time on the planet?

In January, Edward thought about writing a new obituary; he even started one. But for the present, he had put it aside. He seemed to be on the mend again. The mysterious symptoms, the clumsiness, and the gastrointestinal pain were abating, and his T cells had begun to rise again. "It's a big improvement, an enormous improvement," Levinson had said the other night when he gave Edward his new count—378. Edward was much more cautious; 378 was great but only in comparison to 268. In comparison to almost every other number Edward could think of, 378 was terrible.

Besides, overconfidence—any kind of confidence—was dangerous.

AIDS was a great taunter. It would jump out of an alley, scare you silly, then disappear again. This game of hide-and-seek could go on for months, for years, but the end was always the same. When AIDS got tired of toying with your head, it put its hands around your throat and killed you. Edward had seen it happen dozens of times before.

CHAPTER SEVEN

CANDY TALCBUCON WAS SURPRISED.

She had expected the man in the waiting room to be half a head taller and thirty pounds heavier. The voice had fooled her, Candy decided. It was big and booming, so she had assumed that its owner would be, too. Edward Sandisfield was also relatively old, somewhere in his late fifties, and nearly bald—what hair he had left was combed neatly back over a large egg-shaped forehead. There were also small red lesions on his cheeks and forehead. In fact, if you looked quickly you might think Edward was a drinker, but Candy had an experienced eye; she knew the lesions weren't from alcohol.

"Ah, the famous Candy Talcbucon." Edward stood up and smiled.

Edward had wonderful teeth, though. Large, white, and strong-looking. They were easily his best feature, Candy thought.

Edward was surprised at how quiet the trials unit was. The waiting room was empty except for himself and a young black woman reading a copy of *Details*. "Where are the legions of people you've been telling me about?" he asked.

"Things get busy later," Candy said. "It's only eight-thirty."

Edward asked her how many trial spots were available.

"I told you last week . . . twenty-seven."

"And you've reserved one for me, right? I am going to be in this trial." Edward said this in his most stentorian voice.

Candy smiled. "We'll see, Edward, we'll see." Her tone was friendly but noncommittal. "Come with me, please."

The hall outside the waiting room, painted a dull gray-white, ran the length of the building, nearly half a city block. As Edward and Candy walked toward the far end, a door on the left side opened. A young black woman emerged; Edward guessed she was about twenty-two or twenty-three. The doctor with her looked like a rock star. He had long shaggy hair, a Zapata mustache, and a lean Mick Jagger body.

"That's Dr. Gonzalez," Candy said. "He works with Dr. Gulick."

On the right side of the hall there were one, two . . . Edward counted five doors. "The exam rooms," Candy said; she opened the door to the fifth room and gestured to Edward. Inside, there was a man, neatly built and prematurely bald, standing next to an examining table. He walked over and extended his hand when Edward entered.

"Hi, I'm Trip Gulick. Nice to meet you, Mr. Sandisfield. Candy's told me a lot about you."

Edward liked Gulick's face—it was an architect's or a museum curator's face: serious, thoughtful, sensitive. But Gulick was young, to Edward's fifty-four-year-old eyes, very young, and that was worrying; in Edward's experience, young was bad when it came to a clinical trial. Young researchers were interested in building careers and that made them very cautious, very unwilling to take chances. A young researcher was less likely to overlook an infraction of the trial rules, even an innocent one.

Edward opened the manila envelope in his hand and took out a Xerox of his New York State driver's license. He handed it to Dr. Gulick.

The researcher looked surprised. "What's this?"

"Candy said you wanted to see proof of my legal residence."

Candy shrugged and shook her head.

Dr. Gulick handed the Xerox back to Edward. "We don't require proof of residency, Mr. Sandisfield."

"I'm sorry. I must have misunderstood. How thoroughly stupid of me." Edward was blushing.

"That's all right." Dr. Gulick wrote something on a chart, then looked at Edward and smiled. "Is this your first trial, Mr. Sandisfield?"

An official question or was Gulick just making conversation? "I was in a very early AZT trial at St. Luke's–Roosevelt," Edward said, then quickly changed the subject.

"I have something else for you." He opened the envelope and handed Dr. Gulick a second document. This one contained the date, nature, and result of every medical test Edward had taken between April 22, 1992, and February 27, 1995. Dr. Gulick counted forty-three separate tests on the paper. Once he had had a patient who illustrated the changes in his T cell count with colored computer graphics. But he had never seen anything like this before.

"I thought you might find this data useful," Edward said.

Dr. Gulick nodded. "I see you even have footnotes, Mr. Sandisfield."

"Yes, six." Edward pointed a manicured finger at the row of symbols at the bottom of the page. "Mostly, they signify lab errors. You'll see I've dated each one."

The data in Edward's file almost made the purpose of today's physical superfluous. Edward's last set of tests, done on February 27, already provided an up-to-date pretrial or baseline record of his T cell count; viral load; liver, kidney, and heart function; and white and red blood cells.

After the exam, Dr. Gulick asked Edward if he could keep the paper. "It will give us another reference point to measure how the trial drugs affect you."

"Keep it as long as you like," Edward said. He was sitting on the examination table buttoning his shirt. "I have another copy at home."

Dr. Gulick looked down the long rows of neatly printed numbers.

"Mr. Sandisfield."

"Edward, please, Doctor . . ."

"Edward, I don't see a bilirubin count [a measure of liver function] for the twenty-seventh. It should have been in your blood chemistries."

Edward looked at the paper. "How odd. Oh, I see what happened. I forgot to transcribe that reading from my master copy. I'll phone it in to you."

When Dr. Gulick got back to his office later that day, the red light on his answering machine was blinking. He pressed the message button.

"Good afternoon, Dr. Gulick. Edward Sandisfield here. I have that number you wanted. My bilirubin count for the twenty-seventh was point five. If you check it against the January fifth numbers, you'll see a tenth of a percentage increase between the dates. A positive change, I believe."

Dr. Gulick hit the replay button, and leaned back in the chair. The voice on the machine was serious, substantial, intelligent; but it also was engaged in a futile struggle. Dr. Gulick had known patients like Edward before, patients who tried to control their disease with meticulously kept records. The record keeping was a form of magical thinking. Record keepers believed that if you wrote a test result down, it would never change on you, and if the results never changed, you would never get sick and die.

However, Edward's record keeping also suggested conscientiousness and responsibility, two qualities trial 035 would require.

More and more, AIDS was becoming an inner-city disease, and Dr. Gulick wanted trial 035 to reflect the change. He had set aside a third of Bellevue's trial spots for poor and minority patients. But minority patients were often suspicious of doctors, and sometimes the suspicion translated into a tendency to miss appointments, ignore instructions, or drop out of the study. A special support system would be set up to help disadvantaged subjects. Day care would be made available for single mothers, subway and bus fare for poorer subjects. Still, even with these measures, losses were likely. To prevent the dropout rate from becoming unmanageable, trial 035 would need a core group of reliable and conscientious subjects.

Edward was clearly both, and he could be an asset to the trial in another way. He would make a good role model for the other patients. He was obviously well educated, and he possessed a certain self-confidence, a certain weightiness. Dr. Gulick was guessing, but Edward was probably a successful business executive or had been once. He certainly carried himself like someone familiar with authority. Seeing Edward in the elevator or in the waiting room, the poorer subjects might draw a measure of comfort from knowing that AIDS struck the advantaged, too.

"Oh dear, you don't recognize me, do you?"

"Colin?"

"Yes, Colin. Of course, Colin. Edward, how are you? What a delight."

Edward pushed Colin's elegant face from his mind, too early to think about him now. Besides, it would only make the tears start again. Edward got out of bed and walked into the kitchen.

Stephen, his boarder, had forgotten to close the spout on the orange juice again. Edward cursed, snapped the spout shut, and took the milk out of the refrigerator.

Boarders were one of Edward's idiosyncrasies. Lately he had been telling friends that a roommate was an economic necessity; the mortgage payment on the East Seventy-eighth Street co-op could not be met without one. But even when he had had a salary in the mid-six-figure range, Edward had rented out a spare bedroom in the apartment to a succession of graduate students.

Edward poured the milk into his coffee, then walked over to the kitchen window and looked out. He had been in a depression since seeing *Jeffrey* in Miami ten days earlier. In the space of an hour and half, the movie, a comedy of gay life and manners, had managed to remind Edward of every one of the ways HIV had reduced, diminished, isolated, and unmanned him.

Oh, who am I trying to fool? he thought, coming out of the theater that night. Nothing's going to change. Nothing. Even if by some miracle the protease inhibitor worked, it wasn't a magic wand. Edward had hoped New York and the trial would lift his spirits and restore his equilibrium, but then last night at the Townhouse, a favorite watering hole in the East Fifties, Edward had run across another reminder of his former self.

He was sitting at the bar with Lindsay Wilson, an old friend from the Hamptons, when he noticed a dashing-looking middle-aged man with a Guardsman's mustache staring at him. "Laurence Olivier in his Establishment period," Edward said gesturing toward the end of the bar.

Lindsay turned around and looked at the man. "Do you know him?"

"No," Edward said, and ordered another drink.

A few minutes later, Edward felt a finger tapping on his shoulder. When he turned around the man was standing next to him.

"Edward, how are you? It's been what? Nine, no, ten years now."

Edward hesitated.

"Oh dear, you don't recognize me, do you?"

Edward did now. He would recognize that voice anywhere.

Colin was wrong about their last encounter, though. It had been almost twelve years earlier, not ten. Edward remembered the date exactly—June 12, 1983—and he also remembered the circumstances. He had just returned home from a business trip to Europe, had not even been in the door half an hour, when Colin announced in his languid, superior way that he had "a spot of news." While Edward was away, Colin had signed a lease on a new apartment. An hour later he was packed and gone.

It was hard for Edward to connect the suave middle-aged man in front of him with the dark, sensuous, fawnlike creature who had disappeared into the backseat of a cab that night. Colin had been a beautiful young man. Beautiful when they met in Mykonos in 1978, and beautiful when he walked out on Edward five years later. Now Colin looked like a superannuated British colonel up from the Home Counties.

"Are you still at Columbia?" Edward asked.

"Oh dear no, I moved south in 1986. I'm at NYU now."

"Still in art history?"

Colin smiled. "A full professor of art history now."

Oh, that Oxbridge accent, so elegant, so dazzling—so venomous when it chose to be. It was what Edward had fallen in love with first. That voice, that splendid voice, that and Colin's throwaway self-assurance and laconic intelligence. But he turned out to have no heart, no heart at all. Edward gave and Colin received, those were the terms of the relationship. And when Colin got bored with receiving—in truth, got bored with Edward—he had left him.

"Can I buy you and your friend a glass of wine?" Colin smiled at Lindsay.

Edward hesitated. He was surprised at how uncomfortable he felt in Colin's presence, even now, all these years later.

"I have a dinner date at seven-thirty."

Colin looked at his watch. Edward had forgotten what long, graceful hands he had.

"I should think you have time for one drink."

Colin had done quite well for himself, quite well, indeed. A brownstone in the Village, a country house in Stockbridge, a professorship at NYU, and Henry, an investment banker. They had been together now for six years, Colin said. "In fact, we just celebrated our sixth anniversary last month. You must come to dinner one night, Edward. Just the three of us. I know you'll like Henry. He's first-rate, absolutely first-rate."

The Townhouse was on Fifty-eighth Street, but Edward was still crying when he got to Seventy-eighth Street. So he walked over to Central Park, found a bench under a lamppost, and sat there until his tears stopped.

CHAPTER EIGHT

"OH, YOU MEAN THESE."

Miguel Pérez rubbed his finger over the three small purple dots on his chest.

"They're mosquito bites. I got 'em last month."

"They're not mosquito bites."

"No, huh?"

Pérez looked surprised. He was sitting on the edge of the examining table in his Jockey shorts.

"They sure look like mosquito bites, doc." Pérez rubbed his finger over the dots again. He was in his thirties, dark skinned, earringed, and well built. Massively well built. Bowling-ball biceps, wing-sized lats, and a neck like a tree trunk. Probably a bodybuilder.

Trip Gulick took out a penlight and asked Pérez to open his mouth. There were three matching dots inside his mouth on the soft palate.

HIV could be so elusive. The lab tests—and Pérez had completed all fifteen required for trial 035—suggested general good health. Without a physical examination, the low-tech part of the screening process, the dots would have been missed. Dr. Gulick told Pérez he had early stage Kaposi's sarcoma.

"Yeah. I thought it was a little weird, mosquito bites this time of year."

The researcher was surprised. Generally, patients jumped when they heard the word "sarcoma." Pérez didn't seem upset at all.

"That doesn't mean I'm disqualified from the study, does it, doc?"

Dr. Gulick shook his head. "No, early stage KS isn't an exclusion."

"So Pérez stays in the safety study?" Candy asked later that day.

Dr. Gulick nodded. "Pérez stays in. We need every available body."

Pérez along with Edward and ten other men and women selected for the pretrial safety study would be scientific Columbuses—the first human beings to land on planet 035. If the twelve remained healthy and well, on July 11 the FDA would give a final green light, and the other subjects would begin receiving the drugs. If one or more of the twelve became ill or died, planet 035 would be declared a hazard to human life and blown up. The trial would be canceled.

The day of Miguel Pérez's examination, Dr. Gulick's immediate problem was the deadline for the start of the safety study. His hopes of becoming principal investigator for trial 035 rested on his promise to Chodakewitz to have twelve qualified candidates in place and ready by April 28—and the twenty-eighth was only eighteen days away.

In theory, finding twelve physically suited candidates among the hundreds of willing applicants should have been easy. But in practice, the staff did not have hundreds of applicants to choose from; it had only forty. The decision to delay recruitment until the arrival of the final protocol had shortened the screening period to five weeks. And forty was the maximum number of people who could be put through the fifteen-step screening process in five weeks.

The viral-load assay—the first step in the process—immediately eliminated fifteen of the forty candidates. They had either too much or too little virus in their blood. Complete blood counts and chemistries— the second step in the process—eliminated another six, mostly for abnormal liver readings. The liver breaks down drugs, and given the trial drug's toxicity, a healthy liver was an essential requirement. Three other candidates were dropped because of scheduling problems. Two would not be in New York on April 28, the start of the study; the third because his schedule made once-a-week hospital visits impossible.

With the start of the safety study barely two weeks away and the pool of potential subjects down to eighteen, Dr. Gulick was reluctant to lose another candidate, even one with early stage Kaposi's sarcoma. So when Miguel Pérez failed to show up for his next appointment on April 18, the researcher asked Candy to find him. Two phone calls to the Pérez home failed to produce a pickup, so Candy tried his work number. The man who answered the phone told her Miguel had been out sick since the previous Friday. Pérez's aunt, the next person Candy called, didn't know where he was either, but she mentioned a former lover of Pérez's and gave Candy his telephone number. An hour and three phone calls later, a very shaken Pérez was finally tracked down. "Why didn't you come in for your appointment?" Candy asked. Pérez's answer was long and convoluted. But the upshot was that he had gone into hiding.

Four days after the conversation with Dr. Gulick, an emergency room physician at a Bronx hospital had declared the purple dots on Pérez's chest and palate cancerous. Kaposi's sarcoma was an obscure medical term—one of those funny, vague phrases doctors use—but Pérez knew what the word *cancer* meant. He had an aunt and grandfather who had died of the disease—died slow, agonizing deaths. At first, the ER doctor's diagnosis stunned him. Pérez had gone to the hospital expecting to hear that he had a bad flu. Frantic with fear, he considered suicide. The day after the ER visit, he spent an hour pacing back and forth on the Willis Avenue Bridge—one of the bridges that link the boroughs of Manhattan and the Bronx—wondering whether to jump. Next, Pérez decided to go into hiding. Somehow, he got it into his mind that if he hid out he would be safe; and being a native New Yorker, he figured the last place in the world cancer would think to look for him was New Jersey. On April 12, Candy finally tracked Pérez down at his second cousin's house in Weehawken.

In the weeks leading up to April 28, there were several other bizarre and painful encounters with potential subjects.

"You're taking my last chance away," one man told Dr. Gulick on April 12. "My last chance," the man said again and began to cry.

Dr. Gulick knew this candidate was not exaggerating. Indinavir probably was his last chance, but he had only a 46 T cell count and though the trial criteria were flexible enough to admit a sarcoma like Pérez's, Gulick couldn't fudge a T cell count under 50.

Encounters like this one would haunt Dr. Gulick for days. Later, he would think of things he could have said, should have said to rejected candidates. Things that would have made his "no" fall a little more softly on their ears. But so many desperate, beseeching, frightened men and women trooped through his office in late March and early April 1995, it was impossible to find the words to comfort all of them. The researcher was not unaware of the ironic situation 035 had placed him in. In the name of realizing his dream, he was turning away hundreds of desperate people, people in pain, people who were frightened and bewildered, people with parents and children and lovers, people like that young man in the emergency room.

Everyone else on the unit felt the strain too. AIDS was not like other diseases. It was harder for staffers to keep a professional distance. All those sad young faces drew you in, made you angry, broke your heart because they were in such utter misery, and there was so little you could do to help them. Indeed, a recent editorial in *The Archives of General Psychiatry* had worried out loud about the high rate of depression, anxiety, hopelessness, and despair among the doctors and nurses on AIDS units like Bellevue's.

The staff began to take extraordinary measures to accommodate candidates, to give them every possible chance to qualify. Dr. Gulick personally intervened in two cases. One involved a man whose liver reading disqualified him for the trial. Protocol rules said that every candidate got only one liver test. But when the researcher learned that this candidate was on medication at the time of his first test, he ordered Candy to arrange another.

The man's second failure haunted Dr. Gulick for a long time. He felt he'd scheduled the test too soon. The man took it a week after he went off his medication. "I should have made him wait another ten days," Dr. Gulick said later. "A week wasn't enough time for the drug to wash out of his system." Something the candidate's HIV-free lover said after the second test also haunted Dr. Gulick: "We both know Timmy's going to die if he doesn't get these drugs," the lover said. "Put me on the trial and I'll give my drugs to him."

Dr. Gulick had to say no.

The second intervention involved Edward Sandisfield, one of the twelve candidates for the safety trial. The 035 protocol required two pretrial T cell counts from each candidate, and both had to fall within the 50 to 400 range. Edward's first count, 348, was within the designated parameters. But his second, 638, was not; it was an automatic disqualifier.

Oh shit, Edward thought when Candy gave him the second count, the last thing I need now is T cells with a sense of humor. It would take a year of phone calls and letters and flirting and faxes to find another study as good as 035; by that time his 638 count could be back to 268 or maybe lower.

Two days later, in the hall, Dr. Gulick told Edward that one of the counts had to be wrong. The numbers were too far apart. "I told Candy I want you to have another count done." The researcher paused for a moment. "I don't want you to think I'm making an exception for you, Mr. Sandisfield . . ."

"Oh, I don't, Doctor. Edward, please."

"Edward . . . Or that I'm doing you any special favors. I just think an error has been made and I want to rectify it."

Well, who would have thought? Young Dr. Gulick was going to throw him a lifeline, and without any wheedling or pleading from him. Really ... sometimes life could be absolutely astonishing.

Edward smiled all the way down in the elevator.

A week later, the results of the third T cell count came back—398. Two days later, April 26, 1995, Trip Gulick drew up a list of the twelve people who would be the first to step onto planet 035. As a group, they were as diverse as he had hoped they would be. The twelve included:

A fifty-one-year-old Catholic priest (suspected route of HIV infection: sexual contact);

An eighteen-year-old white teenager (suspected route of infection: blood transfusion);

A sixty-three-year-old white grandmother (suspected route of infection: blood transfusion);

A thirty-four-year-old gay Hispanic man (suspected route of infection: sexual contact);

A twenty-four-year-old black mother of two (suspected route of infection: IV drug use);

A nineteen-year-old Asian male (suspected route of infection: multiple sources);

A twenty-eight-year-old Hispanic woman with two children (suspected route of infection: heterosexual sex);

A twenty-four-year-old Hispanic gay man (suspected route of infection: sexual contact);

A twenty-seven-year-old white woman with one child (suspected route of infection: heterosexual sex);

A fifty-year-old Hispanic woman (suspected route of infection: heterosexual sex);

A thirty-two-year-old white gay male (suspected route of infection: sexual contact);

And Edward.

· · ·

Edward was in an ebullient mood today. On his way over to Levinson's office he had stopped at Bellevue and picked up his first supply of drugs. They were inside the brown paper bag—an ordinary number-six lunch bag—in his lap. He held the bag up.

Levinson made an exaggerated bow. "Congratulations, Edward. Really it was an amazing feat; everyone wanted to get into that study. Everyone."

"Thank you, Doctor," Edward said, then got to the reason for his visit. "I have an idea. It's a little . . ." Edward struggled for the right word. He decided on "controversial." Controversial suggested iconoclasm, rather than duplicity. "Please, keep an open mind."

Levinson smiled. "You're talking to Dr. Open Mind."

Edward patted the brown lunch bag and pointed out that while the three vials inside were labeled indinavir, 3TC, and AZT, in actuality, only a third of the subjects were getting the real drugs; the other two-thirds were either getting the protease inhibitor alone, plus two placebos, or 3TC and AZT plus a protease placebo. "The math says I only have a $33^1/3$ percent chance of being in the combination-therapy arm," Edward said.

"And . . ."

"And those are unacceptable odds."

"Everyone in 035 faces the same odds," Levinson noted.

"I know, but that doesn't make them acceptable."

Edward knew how this sounded, but he didn't care. He had known plenty of people who played by the rules, observed study protocols, who did everything their doctors told them to do. Most were dead now. The first law of the jungle he lived in was: If you wanted to live, you had to save your life. No doctor, no researcher, no one else was going to do it for you.

Levinson also knew the rules. He asked Edward what he was proposing.

If he was getting the real indinavir, Edward said, his liver counts and bilirubin readings would shoot up immediately. But AZT and 3TC were difficult to detect in blood chemistries.

Levinson nodded.

Edward said his plan involved a substitution. "If I get the real inhibitor, I want you to write me a prescription for 3TC and AZT."

Levinson asked him what would happen to the AZT and 3TC in the trial packet.

"They go in the wastebasket; I take the real AZT and 3TC you prescribe, plus the real indinavir from the trial. That way, I get the real combination therapy."

Edward said he was sure his plan would not compromise the scientific integrity of the trial. He knew for a fact that study designers always left a statistical margin for schemes like his; they knew cheating went on in AIDS trials. (Like the ddI exclusion, this deception was also unnecessary. Edward, lucky as always, was getting the three real drugs.)

"Well," Edward said, "what do you think?"

Levinson shifted in his chair. He wasn't smiling anymore. "I don't know, Edward."

Edward felt a spike of anxiety. He reminded Levinson of his earlier advice about the study. "You said if necessary, I should 'lie, lie, lie.' "

"I know what I said, Edward, but this is a little different."

"How is this a little different?"

"Well, for one thing, you're in the study now, aren't you?"

Edward was annoyed. "Gulick's job is to worry about the study. Your job is to worry about *me*. We're discussing my life, Sandy. You're my personal physician; your first responsibility is to me."

Levinson put up his hands.

"Enough, please. I am aware of my responsibilities, Edward. Let's wait two months and see if you're getting the real indinavir."

"Then what?"

"Then we'll talk again, is what. I'm not saying no. But you're asking me to do something I'm not entirely comfortable with."

Edward left the meeting upset. Levinson was a good—no, a wonderful—doctor . . . at least, for a certain kind of patient: someone who was already terminally ill and needed a physician with the combined skills of a crisis manager and a Jewish mother. But for someone like himself, for someone who was still relatively healthy and determined to stay that way, Levinson was too passive. He never seemed to have any suggestions beyond "Let's wait two months and see." That's what he'd said the previous fall when the mysterious GI problems developed and what he'd said again last winter when Edward called about the 268 T cell count.

"Do you know what you're going to tell your secretary when I die?" Edward asked during that conversation.

"No," Levinson replied. "What am I going to tell her?"

"You're going to tell her, 'Let's wait two months and see if Edward is really dead.' "

Edward would be the first to admit that he was a demanding patient. He nudged, he bullied, he complained and whined. He wanted to know the reason for every medical decision and he wanted an explanation for every item on every bill. Above all, he wanted aggressiveness.

"Jesus," Levinson had exploded the previous month when Edward presented him with a ten-point discussion list, "do you ever let up?" Edward said no and pushed the list over to Levinson's side of the desk. If you wanted to live, you had to be as relentless as the virus, and sometimes as amoral, too. As he was leaving today, Edward told Levinson he could have four weeks to think about the plan, "then we'll discuss it again. Adieu, Sandy."

When he got home, Edward took a bottle of Tanqueray gin down from the liquor cabinet, walked into the kitchen and opened the cabinet over the kitchen sink. "Damn, no glasses." Stephen never put anything away. Edward removed a dirty glass from the dishwasher, rinsed it out in the sink, then picked up the bottle of Tanqueray from the kitchen counter and filled the glass halfway with gin.

He took a sip and walked over to the answering machine in the hall. The message light was blinking. Edward pushed the replay button. One, two, three . . . he counted to thirty before the cackling tape finally stopped rewinding. He must have at least two messages.

The first was from Jonathan Applecroft.

Jonathan was a relatively new friend. Edward had met him and his lover David Evans last winter in Key West. They were two blue-eyed, chiseled-featured, handsome young Wall Streeters. Two matching bookends—one blond, one redheaded—who, between them, made more than a million dollars a year. Now, barring a miracle, one member of this golden couple was going to die. Last night, an ambulance had taken the younger one, David, to Columbia-Presbyterian.

"David's got PCP again," Jonathan's message said.

The news did not come as a complete surprise. Last week at the Townhouse, Jonathan said that David was having night sweats again. In the early years of the epidemic, PCP was almost always fatal—less so now. But David, stricken with PCP twice already, was not likely to survive a third bout.

Edward wondered how David's parents, evangelical Christians, would take the news. David had told them he was HIV positive only four months before. Corky's theory was that waiting until the end was the worst thing you could do to a parent. A parent needed time to adjust to the thought of your death.

The other messages contained better news.

The first was from Levinson. He apologized for being so negative this morning. As soon as they knew what arm of the study Edward was in, they could discuss the substitution plan again.

The last message, from Corky, was congratulatory.

"Good for you, Mr. Sandisfield. Quite a coup, getting into that study. You're a rare and splendid fellow."

"Gorgeous, too," Edward told the machine. He was surprised at how happy he felt. "Watch that, mister," he told himself. Hope was a dangerous thing; it could always turn around and bite you later. Edward walked back into the kitchen and picked up his study bag. He put down his gin, and opened the bag. There was a second clear plastic bag inside. The tag on it said:

Trial: 035
Drugs: MK 69281 (Indinavir)
MK 4920 (AZT)
MK 13334 (3TC)
Patient ID: #211
Patient's name: Edward Sandisfield

Edward was surprised to find his name on the tag. Only ID numbers were supposed to be used in HIV studies. What was wrong with Merck? What if the bag got lost or stolen? God knows where his name would end up. Edward ripped the tag off, tore it up, and threw the pieces in the wastebasket. Including Gulick, Candy, and Gonzalez, only eight people in the world knew he was HIV positive and he intended to keep it that way.

There were three vials inside the plastic bag. Edward removed the one marked MK 4920. The small red-and-white AZT capsules inside were different from commercial AZT tablets. A researcher Edward knew said that this was a security measure. In the late 1980s, when AZT was *the* hot new AIDS agent, some trial subjects had sold their study supply on the street. Pharmaceutical companies had switched to a different-type tablet to make street sales easier to track.

The tablets inside the indinavir and 3TC vials were beige and much larger. Underneath the vials, Edward found a slip of paper with dosage instructions. The drugs were to be taken in the following combinations at eight-hour intervals:

Morning: AZT, 3TC, indinavir.
Afternoon: AZT, indinavir
Evening: AZT, 3TC, indinavir

Edward smiled when he read that alcohol was a contraindication. Over the years, he had taken thousands of pills while also enjoying a few daily doses of gin. This had greatly offended his first HIV doctor,

Michael Tollard.* "How can you drink like you do and take AZT?" an outraged Tollard had said to him once.

"It's easy," Edward told him.

Levinson, who worried about everything, also worried about Edward's drinking. But Edward, so careful about his health in other ways, refused to give up alcohol. It was his last connection to normal life and he intended to keep it. Whenever he began to feel guilty about his drinking, he reminded himself that sobriety had not done the HIV-positive Dr. Tollard any good. He was dead now.

Edward poured a little more gin into his glass and then removed a pill from each vial and lined them up next to one another on the kitchen counter. They certainly were an unprepossessing-looking lot. No superpills here, Edward thought; he could be looking at a collection of diet pills. One by one, Edward put the tablets in his mouth, took a large swig of gin, and swallowed. Then he walked back into the living room and picked up the TV remote from the couch. He pressed the on button; the long, bony face of the young Fred Astaire appeared on the television screen. AMC (American Movie Channel) was replaying the old Astaire–Ginger Rogers classic *Swing Time* again this afternoon. Edward had watched the movie last night. He had come in on the gazebo scene. Fred Astaire was just beginning to sing:

Isn't it a lovely day.
Isn't it a lovely day to be caught in the rain.

Edward began to hum along.

Isn't it a lovely day to be all cozy and warm.

Fred and Ginger were dancing now, gliding across the gazebo. Edward began to glide along with them.

*Pseudonym

CHAPTER NINE

A FEW WEEKS BEFORE TRIAL 035 BEGAN, FIVE PATIENTS DIED SUD-
denly in a hepatitis B trial. News of the tragedy served to underscore
what everyone at the Bellevue trials unit already knew: Even with animal data and computer simulations, even with data from other human
studies, once a new drug or a new drug combination enters the human body, it is impossible to predict what will happen. On April 27,
Dr. Gulick warned the unit staff to be prepared for anything because
anything could happen now. But no one, including Dr. Gulick, expected what did happen: nothing. Absolutely nothing. There were no
complaints about tiredness, GI distress, headaches—no complaints
about any of the common, garden-variety little ills that people normally
complain about at the start of a new trial. Everyone in trial 035 felt
good, and in some cases, more than good. "Yesterday," one excited man
told Candy, "I cleaned my apartment, cooked a meal for six, and stayed
up until two A.M. talking. I haven't had this much energy in years." Another subject spent the weekend gardening, something she had long
been unable to do.

"It's the placebo effect," Dr. Gulick told himself. People always got euphoric at the start of a trial. It was human nature. Hope always won out, at least for a while. Still, something more than hope was clearly at work in the T cells of Paul O'Dell. A tall, gangly Howard Stern look-alike, O'Dell appeared for his first interview at the trials unit dressed like the Biker from Hell; for his first blood test, like the Marlboro Man, and for his physical, like the commander of the SS *Montana*.

O'Dell's real life was not nearly as vivid as his imagination. He was a hairdresser, and despite his taste for over-the-top macho dress, a surprisingly gentle soul. He also was the first person in 035 to experience a hundred-point T cell gain.

A week after O'Dell's count shot up, Ti Chaun Kaun's followed suit.

Ti was known to the trial staff as "Mr. Everything," a nickname he received from Candy at the intake interview. Candy ran down the list of possible HIV infection sources and then, Ti, a model of Asian politeness, bowed deeply and replied, "Everything." Ti said he'd had sex with men and sex with women; sex with male prostitutes and sex with female prostitutes; he had been an intravenous drug user and had had blood transfusions up and down the Pacific Rim, in the United States, and in China and in the Philippines.

Several other subjects, including Edward, showed a different response pattern. On April 26, Edward's T cell count was 422; on June 7, nearly five weeks later, still 422. But then it rose abruptly. On June 21, Dr. Gonzalez announced with much fanfare that Edward's T cell count was 611.

Gonzalez looked a little disappointed when his patient shrugged. "I thought you'd be excited," the physician said.

"Counts jump up and down," Edward replied. "Tomorrow, it could be two sixty-eight again."

Edward truly believed this, but in the early summer of 1995 his behavior suggested that, slowly and cautiously, he was beginning to believe something else, too. He might have a few more good years of life left, after all. The first part of Edward to react to this unexpected news was his libido. Edward's last real romance, a 1990 affair with a young Finnish painter in Paris, had ended in a traumatic dream. In the dream, he and the painter, a young man named Stefan, were standing alone in a large, empty room. "Go away, I'm infected," Edward shouted across the room. But Stefan either did not hear the warning or did not care. He began to walk toward Edward. "Go away," Edward shouted again. "Go away." But it was too late. Stefan reached out and touched him. The last thing Edward remembers before he woke up was the painter lying dead on the floor in front of him.

The next day, the day he had planned to tell Stefan he was HIV positive, Edward suddenly announced that he had to return to New York on business. "But you can't," Stefan protested. Edward had promised to fly up to Helsinki that weekend for an exhibition of Stefan's paintings.

"I have to," Edward said. "I have no choice."

After Stefan, Edward's sex life had more or less ended. He decided that he would never expose himself to that kind of pain again. But now suddenly, after a four-year interval of celibacy, he found himself noticing attractive men on the street again and, surprise of surprises, fantasizing about sex. One Sunday afternoon, he even let Alan Gillis talk him into a Body Positive Tea Dance at GMHC. Did these changes mean that he had stopped thinking of himself as a condemned man? "No," Edward told himself. But more and more, Edward's behavior suggested yes.

In late June, Edward decided to do something about a long-standing sexual problem. "I don't know whether it's age or the medications," Edward told Levinson one muggy afternoon, "but I haven't had an erection for two years."

"That's a long time, Edward."

"I know it's a long time, Sandy. What can we do about it?"

"Testosterone therapy," Levinson said. "I'm going to put you on testosterone therapy."

Edward also consulted his New York dermatologist, Michael Cronin.* Cronin, a tall, flamboyant man with the ruined good looks of a Peter O'Toole, was Edward's favorite doctor—possibly because Cronin, alone among his doctors, did not scold him for drinking too much. Once, when Edward worried out loud about his alcohol consumption, Cronin waved his arm dismissively in the air, and said in a deep, leading-man voice, "Edward, an alcoholic is someone who drinks more than his doctor; you, dear boy, have a long way to go."

Thirty years of too much sun had aged Edward's skin prematurely. Would a chemical peel help shave off a few years? he asked Cronin.

"Help?" Cronin said, suddenly as fluttery as Big Bird. "Help? It'll do more than help. You'll be gorgeous."

The trials unit staff also noticed a change in Edward. At the beginning of the study, no one called the unit as much as he did. Mostly, Edward's calls were about details only Edward would notice. Why was his bilirubin level up a half a point this week? Why was his cretin level down half a point? When was Merck going to stop putting his name on the test drugs? If Dr. Gulick was unavailable, Edward would call Candy, and if Candy was unavailable, he would call Dr. Gulick. And he would always leave a long, detailed message with each.

For a while, "Hello, Edward Sandisfield here . . ." became as much a part of their day as the rumble of traffic outside on First Avenue. But sometime in the middle of July, Edward began to call less. "I wonder why?" Candy said one day.

Dr. Gulick didn't offer an opinion, but he thought he knew why. Edward was becoming less afraid.

During the first three months of the study, only two things disturbed Edward's peace of mind. One was Levinson's backpedaling about the AZT and 3TC prescriptions.

*Pseudonym

"It's still too early," he told Edward one afternoon in early July. "We don't know if you're on indinavir yet." Edward started to argue, but Levinson cut him off. "We'll talk again in August," he said.

A week later, David Evans died. The death was not unexpected, but the incident that followed it left Edward upset for weeks. David's parents wanted Jonathan, David's lover and the executor of his will, to allot a portion of the $40,000 bequest David had made to GMHC to the family's church—to the church David was baptized and brought up in.

But Jonathan refused; he told them he felt honor bound to carry out David's wishes.

The incident occurred the afternoon of the funeral. According to Corky, who told Edward about it the next day, after the family came back from the cemetery, David's mother went "berserk" in Jonathan's apartment. She accused him of turning David into a homosexual. Then she threw a vase at him and called him a "filthy murderer."

Corky's news didn't entirely surprise Edward. David's mother had thrown herself on the casket as it was being lifted into the hearse.

"Jonathan should have given part of the GMHC money to the family's church," Edward said. "He was asking for trouble, being that rigid."

"Jesus, Edward, you really do reduce everything to money, don't you?" Corky sounded exasperated. "David's mother went nuts because David was selfish. He didn't want to deal with her pain, so he didn't tell her he was positive until five months ago. He didn't give her enough time to prepare herself. The money was just a trigger. If it hadn't been the bequest, something else would have set her off." Corky paused. "I know it's an old song, Edward, but you really ought to tell Evelyn. It'll be ten times harder on her if you wait until the end."

Edward was beginning to think that there was not going to be an end—not soon, anyway. But he didn't tell Corky that. He just said, "Maybe. Let me think about it."

A few days after this conversation, Dr. Gonzalez called with the results of Edward's latest T cell test. They were not good. Edward's count had tumbled nearly 400 points in under a month—from 605 to 248. "You should have another test done as soon as possible," Gonzalez told him.

"I'll be in in the morning," Edward said.

CHAPTER TEN

Right after his diagnosis, a friend told Edward that the worst part of being HIV positive was the uncertainty. AIDS was a strange disease, the friend said; often the symptoms came and went without rhyme or reason, and they had a maddening unspecificity. They could be caused by a lot of things, including innocent things, like colds, stress, tiredness, food, drugs, or your own paranoia. With HIV, the friend warned, you could never be sure what was real and what was not, what was safe and what could kill you.

In the fall of 1995, Edward, already used to uncertainty, encountered profound uncertainty.

Initially, the precipitous drop in his T cell count seemed to have a simple explanation. A technical error. The main lab at NYU was closed down for vacation in August, so Edward's blood sample had been sent to a VA lab in the Bronx for analysis. Everyone in the trials unit was sure that the VA lab had screwed up. Edward's new test would produce a higher count.

"Two seventy-eight!" Edward said a week later, when the new count came back. "How can that be? The count's barely budged."

"Probably another lab error," Dr. Gulick said. "We had to use the Bronx VA again; NYU is still closed. If I were you, I'd discount both readings, Edward. Forget about them."

Medicine mystified Edward.

In the real world, the world uncushioned by tenure and research grants, you could be fired for sending a second sample to a lab that had screwed up the first. But in medicine, at least in the part of medicine Edward was familiar with, screwups seemed to have no consequences. People just kept sending samples off until the lab got it right or the patient dropped dead of anxiety.

Still, Gulick was right about the counts, Edward thought. They should be dismissed, forgotten. You couldn't let a stupid lab error destroy your sanity. Who knows what had gone wrong? A phone call, a hangover—a million things could have distracted the lab technician who analyzed his count. The medical system puts you at the mercy of all sorts of freak accidents. There was also another reason to dismiss the 278, Edward reminded himself: no symptoms. Last December, when his count dropped to 268, he had felt sick and looked sick. Now he felt fine.

A week after the second T cell count came back, Edward drove out to Southampton to shut down the cottage he had rented for the summer. After a quiet dinner in front of the television, Edward took out a pencil and paper and made a "To Do" list for the next day: call the cleaning lady, pack up the dishes, wineglasses, and linens, drop by the butcher's in Amagansett and settle the August bill. At 11:30, after being promised a crisp, cool early autumn weekend by the manically cheerful Al Roker, Edward shut off the TV, turned down the thermostat, and laid out his clothes: a light gray wool sweater and a new pair of slacks from Saks. Then he went to bed.

Edward awoke at 3:05. He remembers the time exactly because the only light in the bedroom came from the bright green numbers on the digital clock. He also remembers noticing the wetness immediately. The bed. The pillow. The sheets, the blanket, everything was dripping wet. Edward turned the night-light on. The top and bottom sheets were soaked through; there was also a sticky film of perspiration over his arms, chest, and legs.

A night sweat!

Edward waited for the sour little pricks of anxiety to subside, then got up, went into the bathroom, and stripped. In the shower, he remembered seeing a thermometer in the medicine cabinet. He took his temperature while he was toweling off. Normal, 98.1; he put the thermometer back and went into the bedroom. A thick, musky scent hung over everything. After he changed the sheets, Edward sprayed the room with Glade, then went into the kitchen, turned on the light, and sat down.

What did he really know? He knew that two conditions associated with full-blown AIDS, PCP, or *Pneumocystis carinii* pneumonia, and MAC, or *Mycobacterium avium* complex, could produce night sweats. But PCP and MAC infections also produced other symptoms, and Edward had no other symptoms, not unless you wanted to count a slight weight loss. No cough, no weakness, no fever. Therefore, Edward decided, it would be rational to consider another less alarming explanation for the sweat. The sheets on the bed were polyester and polyester does not breathe. A warm night, a warm bedroom, a barely opened window, sheets that do not breathe—it was well within the realm of possibility that this peculiar combination of circumstances could have produced the sweat.

Ten days later, Levinson announced that he would not give Edward prescriptions for AZT and 3TC. His no was very gentle. He told Edward that they both wanted the same thing: Edward's health and well-being. But, he said, why prescribe the drugs when Edward's test results strongly suggested he was already getting them?

Edward started to argue. In the spring, hadn't the two of them agreed that it was impossible to detect AZT and 3TC from lab readings?

But this time, Levinson refused to be intimidated. "Throwing away perfectly good drugs is criminal," he said. "I'm not going to be a party to it, Edward. Sorry."

At the end of September, Edward had another night sweat. But this time only the pillowcase and the neck of his T-shirt got wet. After he sponged off, Edward took his temperature—98.1. Normal again. He went out to the linen closet in the hall. HIV patients always assumed the worst when something happened. But you had to look at the big picture, Edward reminded himself, as he removed a set of fresh sheets from the closet. And there was much in his big picture to feel reassured about. There was his new T cell count, 511, and there were the steroids. A few weeks ago, Levinson had told him that night sweats were a common side effect of steroids.

"You probably had a reaction to the injections you got in August for your back," Levinson said.

Edward expressed surprise. "I would never have put the two together."

"See, Edward? You're always so quick to catastrophize."

Levinson, however, turned out to be only half right about the steroids. They could cause night sweats, but, according to Edward's back doctor, just for a few days after an injection. Edward's last injection had been a long time ago—August 18. Conceivably, it could have caused the first sweat, but not the second, or the third, which occurred on October 11.

The evening after the third sweat, Edward began leaving a thermometer on his nightstand. At first, its presence bothered him; he was conceding that the sweats were now permanent, not transitory. But prudence won out. Getting an accurate temperature reading during a sweat was important; a thermometer on the night table would allow Edward to take his temperature the moment he awoke.

Toward the end of October, Edward also gave up trying to explain away the sweats. It required too much energy; anyway, it was futile. He sweated as heavily on cotton sheets as he did on polyester, and he sweated as heavily now as he had in early September after the steroid shots. Possibly, maybe even probably, the sweats were HIV related. But Edward, the contextualizer, told himself that the sweats had to be seen in context to be understood. Night sweats might have sent Jack Scarf home to Oklahoma to die and shrunk big, hulking David Evans down to a quivering 138 pounds. But the *experts*, the Levinsons and Gonzalezes and Gulicks, seemed to regard Edward's sweats more as background noise from HIV than as anything deadly. If the experts were not alarmed, why should he be?

One Sunday, Edward decided to analyze his T cell counts from trial 035. The results were surprising: despite five months of wild ups and downs, Edward's *average* study count was only twenty-two points higher than his average prestudy count. Edward was sure a comparison of his study and prestudy viral assays (the study assays were blind for everyone in 035 but Emilio Emini and his group) would also show little or no change.

But Edward was wrong. His Merck file, the file of patient 211, shows that in late October 1995 the amount of HIV in Edward's blood (what an assay measures) was approaching the undetectable level. The puzzling group of symptoms Edward experienced in the fall of 1995 may have been caused by microscopic amounts of virus (with wily HIV, always a possibility), by Edward's imagination (also always a possibility), or by an unrelated condition.

On October 30, the woman who cleaned Edward's South Beach apartment called. She wanted to know when he was coming down. Edward paused for a moment. He had almost no friends left in Miami; if he left New York in early November, he would end up spending Thanksgiving alone. On the other hand, did he really want to linger in the city just for the sake of a Thanksgiving dinner with friends? The autumn had been awful, brutal; one thing after another. "I'll be down on the eighteenth," he told the woman.

The evening before Edward left for Miami, Michael, Corky's lover, phoned. He told Edward that he had just rushed Corky to the ER of a local hospital. "It was really scary," Michael said. "Corky began getting these awful chest pains at dinner. I thought he was going to die."

Poor Corky, Edward thought. Wan little Michael was the last person in the world he would want to get sick around.

"Do they know what it is yet, Michael?"

"They think it might be a heart attack. As soon as I know more, I'll call you."

As Edward hung up, Robert Novak was pointing a stubby finger at Michael Kinsley on *Crossfire*.

Edward shut off the television and walked over to the window. Corky, he thought, would outlast everyone; would outlast him, anyway. More and more, life was beginning to resemble a game of Ten Little Indians, and now he was the last one left standing. Edward pulled back the curtain and looked down. Ricardo the doorman was standing under a lamppost, talking to Stephen; Stephen was late with the rent again. Edward looked down at his boarder for a moment, then went back to the bedroom and finished packing.

Thanksgiving Day in Miami was unseasonably cool. It was 51 degrees when Edward woke up, and the radio was predicting a high only in the low sixties. At 9:30, Manuel the gardener buzzed. "I'm in the lobby, Meester Sandisfield," he shouted into the intercom. What was Manuel doing here? Edward wondered, then remembered, Manuel was Guatemalan; Thanksgiving was just another workday to him. Edward felt a surge of gratitude as he pressed the door button. Talkative Manuel would make the morning go quicker.

In the early afternoon, Edward went to a movie at a multiplex in Miami City. When he got home, he thought about calling Evelyn. She would be at Darryl's today; so would Tom. The whole family would be at Darryl's for Thanksgiving. But if anyone called anyone today, Edward felt, it should be the Sandisfields who called *him*. He put a Stouffer's chicken pot pie in the microwave, then went into the living room to lie down until it was ready. The 1,500-mile drive from New York had exhausted him.

Last night, Michael had called to say that Corky was all right. Muscle spasms—not, as the doctors had first feared, a heart attack—were responsible for the chest pains. There was also another happy development: Edward's night sweats had disappeared. But Edward was still very concerned about his health. The other day, stepping into the elevator, he thought he noticed a new symptom, a weakness in his right leg. The sensation was so fleeting—no longer than a breath, really—that he could not be sure. The weakness could have been real or it could have been a figment of Edward's aroused imagination.

In late November, there were a half dozen other ambiguous incidents. One morning, reaching for his glasses, Edward hit the lamp on the bedstand. Two days later, walking out to the terrace, he noticed a slight hesitation in his gait. Was he imagining that, too? Edward turned around and walked into the living room again. No, his right leg was moving a fraction slower than his left.

Finally, on December 1, something truly frightening happened. Edward was in bed, reading, when his legs suddenly began to tremble. He ripped off the top sheet, put a hand on each knee and pressed hard. No good. The shaking continued. Next, Edward tried tucking his legs up under his chin and holding them with his arms. That worked. Edward counted to twenty, then relaxed his grip. No movement; the legs remained still. But Edward was afraid to move; he sat on the bed hugging himself until his heart stopped pounding.

The next morning, the weakness in the right leg returned, but this time it did not disappear immediately. It lingered for a day and then another day. There were also several new trembling incidents. Mostly they involved the legs, but once, reaching to pick up his shoes, Edward's left arm began to shake. In addition, he was having at least one "accident" a day now, sometimes two. He was dropping glasses or hitting things. The mysterious gastrointestinal discomfort of the year before also reappeared. Edward felt bloated all the time now. Each day, from December first through the seventh, at least one new symptom appeared.

Later, trying to describe this period to a friend, Edward compared it to having the floor open up underneath you. As each new symptom appeared, Edward would sway this way, then that, trying to maintain his balance, but he was sure that very soon—in a day, in a week at most—the gap in the floor would be too wide to straddle. Then he would fall into the pit below: A full-blown episode of AIDS or something worse. But on December eighth, the floor suddenly stopped moving; no new symptoms appeared. Then on the ninth, inexplicably, the floor began to close up. The first symptom to abate was the trembling, then the gastrointestinal distress, then, finally, the weakness.

CHAPTER ELEVEN

By early December 1995, Dr. Gulick had noticed three distinct response patterns among 035 subjects; some, like Paul O'Dell, responded immediately and dramatically to the trial regimen; others, like Edward, responded more slowly, but also dramatically. In December, Edward's T cell count was 700—higher than it had been in years. A third group of subjects had a bell-shaped response; an initial rise, then a decline.

Overall, these patterns were exciting; the slow and fast responders accounted for 70 percent of the patients in 035, and their average T cell gain was over 100 points. But in mid-December, Dr. Gulick learned that even more exciting news was in the offing. On the fifteenth, Jeff Chodakewitz called and told him that Merck had decided to lift its embargo on the viral-assay results. Chodakewitz said he would reveal the results to the four on-site investigators on the twenty-first during a conference call. Dr. Gulick hung up, excited. He knew Merck would not break the embargo unless there was something very good to reveal.

And, indeed, there was.

At the start of the conference call, Chodakewitz announced that 85 percent of the subjects in the 035 treatment arm—that is, more than four-fifths of the patients receiving the three real drugs—no longer had detectable HIV in their blood. Undetectable isn't the same as virus-free—current assay techniques cannot detect very low levels of HIV—but this result was nonetheless spectacular. Never before had a therapy made the virus disappear.

Chodakewitz waited for everyone to absorb the good news, then he said that the T cell gains in the protease-inhibitor-alone group matched those of subjects in the combination group—an average rise of 100 points or more. But he said that the viral-assay results in the indinavir-alone group were less encouraging. Sixty percent of the subjects still had detectable HIV in their blood, and in the 3TC-AZT group, everyone still did. These differences raised troubling ethical questions. Chodakewitz said he did not think trial 035 could continue in its present form.

The four on-site investigators agreed. After some discussion, they also agreed that the combination therapy—the indinavir, AZT, and 3TC—should be made available to all 035 subjects for the remainder of the study.

There was also unanimity on another point: The viral-load results should be reported immediately. But where? Chodakewitz said the best and most immediate venue would be the National AIDS Conference in February. Everyone on the conference call knew that the person who presented the assay data at the meeting would become an instant medical celebrity. Chodakewitz asked the on-site investigators who they thought should present the results.

Dr. Joseph Eron of the University of North Carolina said, "It should be Trip." Chodakewitz paused for a moment, then said, "Joe's right. Trip's the lead investigator on this study. He should make the presentation."

· · ·

"Come. Christmas in Connecticut."

"I'd rather spend Christmas in a bathing suit."

"You'll spend Christmas at a movie, Edward. You, me, and Michael; it'll be fun. We'll build a snowman."

Edward said it was not supposed to snow.

"So I'll buy an extra bottle of gin. If it doesn't snow, we'll have something to console ourselves with."

"All right, Corky," Edward said, "I'll give you the gift of my person for Christmas."

Edward's train pulled into the Cos Cob station at 10 A.M., Christmas morning. Standing on the platform in the thin winter light, honking, ruddy, boundlessly confident Corky looked gray and old and uncertain. Corky's T cell count had been under 400 since the summer of 1991, four and a half years, a long time to have the virus eating away at you. And now the chest pains. The chest pains must have really frightened Corky, Edward thought. Corky was so greedy for life.

"Well, don't you look pretty, Mr. Sandisfield."

Edward was standing on the platform now with his overnight bag. He smiled at Corky. "Pretty is as pretty does. That's what Evelyn always says."

"Well, if anyone would know, it's our Evelyn, isn't it?" Corky embraced Edward. "Nice to see you again, old thing."

There was no snow in Connecticut, but there was plenty of gin and a big Christmas tree—an enormous Christmas tree. Michael, who seemed very proud of the tree, told Edward that it was over nine feet tall; it had taken him and Corky nearly an hour to get it into the house and another hour to decorate it.

After lunch, Corky and Edward drove over to the Cos Cob shore. On the water, the air was biting, and very cold, but bracing, and the beach was wonderfully still. Only the crunch of sand underfoot and the occasional caw of a passing seagull broke the quiet. Around four, as the Long Island Sound began to swallow up a dull winter sun, Corky drove them back to the house and a big, gossipy Christmas dinner prepared by Michael. It was attended by a dozen mutual friends, most of whom worked at the AIDS hospice Corky had cofounded. At nine, when everyone had gone, Corky slipped *Christmas in Connecticut* into the VCR. He and Edward watched it twice.

Sometimes after a day like this one, after a day this good, Edward would begin to fantasize about normal life, about what it would be like to have a happy day and not have to put an asterisk next to it, not have to remind yourself that this could be the last one. Usually, after a minute or two, Edward would force himself back to the real world, to the world of viruses and drugs and pain and death. But tonight, undressing in Corky's guest room, he felt his discipline slipping. There was a buzz in the air about the trial. People were saying that the combination therapy might be it, the one; it might not just buy a few extra years of life, it might buy something like normal life.

In early January, an air of expectation and excitement spread through the clinical trials unit. Patients, doctors, nurses, everyone knew that Dr. Gulick would be giving a speech about trial 035 on February 6, and everyone sensed that he was going to say something important, something that could change lives. But at the end of January, Jeff Chodakewitz called again.

He said Emilio Emini would give a lecture on protease inhibitors on the opening day of the AIDS conference, Monday, February 2. Emini planned to use a finding from 035 in his talk.

Dr. Gulick asked which finding.

The assay results, Chodakewitz said.

This was the most dramatic and newsworthy result in 035. Emini's announcement would reduce Gulick's talk on the sixth to a postscript, to yesterday's news.

"Drug companies do this kind of thing all the time," Fred Valentine, Dr. Gulick's boss, told him few days after the Chodakewitz call. "I know you feel disappointed. But you're still the lead investigator on the study. In terms of your career here, at NYU, that's what counts. The other stuff is just showbiz."

On February 7, Dr. Gulick returned from the AIDS conference to an answering machine full of congratulatory messages. But the message that caught his attention was left by someone he did not know, a Mrs. Edith Starkwell of Louisiana. Mrs. Starkwell said that she had read about Dr. Gulick and a new AIDS drug in a local paper. (Several of the wire services had covered his speech on the sixth.) She wanted to get more information about the drug. On the machine, her voice sounded back-country southern and desperate.

"I want it for Billy, my son," Mrs. Starkwell said when Dr. Gulick called the number she left. Billy, she explained, was her oldest boy; he was twenty and he was lying in the next room now, dying of AIDS.

Dr. Gulick knew enough other "Billys" to fill in the blanks. Billy had probably contracted AIDS hustling or doing drugs in some big city; when he got too sick to care for himself, he'd come home to his mother and the godforsaken trailer park he couldn't wait to escape. Now Billy was probably going to die in the park.

"He's in awful agony, doctor." Edith Starkwell sounded bewildered, bewildered the way medieval peasants must have been bewildered by the Black Death; she had no idea what AIDS was or how you got it, all she knew was that the disease was killing her son and killing him in a horrible way.

Dr. Gulick promised Mrs. Starkwell he would find a protease inhibitor study for her Billy.

Edward, who followed the conference with great interest from South Beach, had conflicting feelings when he read a report about Dr. Gulick's speech in the *Miami Herald* on February 7. Edward supposed that he was now officially a beneficiary of every sick person's dream—

a real, an authentic lifesaving medical breakthrough. But Edward, an expert in ferreting out hidden downsides, saw several hidden downsides in this unexpected development.

The journey to death is usually described as a descent, but Edward had found it more an ascent; at the top step, the step just below the door marked EVERMORE, he thought the view wonderfully good. From the next-to-the-last step, you could see the harried, frantic, antlike masses scurrying about beneath you, worrying about mortgages and sex and four-wheel drives and face-lifts and what parties they were invited to in the Hamptons. You could see how silly and stupidly they behaved and, almost as good, how silly and stupidly you used to behave when you were an ant. More life would mean becoming an ant again.

More life would also mean more Edward; and Edward was a surly, greedy, appallingly demanding companion. He was a bundle of quivering appetites, appetites that were becoming harder and harder for the aging Edward to fill. Besides, even if he lived an extra thousand years, Edward would always behave in the same old predictable Edward ways. It would be nice to be free of him, to be something else for a change. Sometimes Edward fantasized about becoming light, light the color of a brilliant July sun. Light was beautiful and eternal and it never felt any pain.

More life would also mean old age; and old age meant becoming one of those old fags at the Townhouse, the ones who still primped and preened two hours a day out of habit, who dressed for one another now, because no one else cared.

On the other hand . . .

More life would also mean more time with the people he loved, more time with Corky and Levinson and Evelyn, although, God knows, she was her own one-woman health hazard. It would also mean not having to put an asterisk next to every good day, at least not for another ten or fifteen years; it would mean being able to plan a trip without wondering whether you would be too sick to go; it would mean the possibility of another Colin; and it would mean no more dreams about walking through fire, or worries about what the Seattle Sandisfields would be told, or whether nervous Levinson would panic and execute the living will too soon. It would mean walking out the door on a balmy February morning like this one, and strolling down Collins Avenue without a thought in your head, except the baguette you would bring back for lunch.

Edward had not taken a walk like that in almost seven years. He put the paper down and put on his jacket.

POSTSCRIPT

FIVE WEEKS LATER, MARCH 14, 1996, INDINAVIR WAS APPROVED BY the Food and Drug Administration, the fastest approval time in FDA history. In the last two years, indinavir and other protease inhibitors have changed the face of AIDS treatment. Thousands of patients who otherwise might not be alive are alive because of the combination therapy tested in trial 035. However, in the spring and summer of 1997, follow-up studies began to pick up reports of treatment failure, cases where the therapy failed to beat back the virus.

"There is a growing sense that combination therapies do not succeed in all patients," says Dr. Gulick. The researcher blames some of the failures on the complexity of the combination regimens: the treatment schedule—three drugs taken in different combinations several times daily—can easily confuse a patient. In other cases, he believes, combination therapies fail because patients go on them sequentially. They start with one drug, add a second a month later, and a third a month after that. "Combination treatments work best when all three drugs are taken at once," Dr. Gulick says.

According to the researcher, many of the reports of drug resistance that have surfaced among protease patients are linked to one or both of these sources. He says that researchers are currently working on ways to simplify the combination regimens and to develop new ways to help patients who have become resistant to them.

Thus far, Edward and Corky, who recently began taking the protease inhibitor "cocktail," have not encountered any resistance problems. They continue to do well.

ROMY'S
KNEE

CHAPTER ONE

ONE OF THE GREAT MYSTERIES ABOUT ROMY'S KNEE IS WHY IT WORKED AT a McDonald's on the New Jersey Turnpike at four in the afternoon, but not two and half hours later in Smithtown, Long Island. What happened in those hours? Did the knee simply weary of Romy—grow tired of carrying her up and down, here and there? Or did the cancer finally overwhelm some last defense line? Even today, after four oncologists, five surgeons, fourteen bone scans, two operations, 280 days of hospitalization, half a million dollars in medical bills, after all that and more, no one knows for sure.

Romy Meaghann Hochman was born at Sibley Memorial Hospital in Washington, D.C., on March 2, 1980. About her first hometown, Laurel, Maryland, Romy remembers little except that all the houses looked alike and everyone in town, including her father, Jack, worked for the government. Romy also remembers little about her early life, except that at some point her father stopped commuting to Washington, where he had been a senior government health analyst, and started commuting to Bethesda, where he bought a TCBY (The Country's Best Yogurt) franchise. Romy also remembers that sometime during the Laurel years her mother, Pam, stopped seeming like her mother. Mostly, Romy says, this was because Pam was never around. Pam, who had a serious drug problem, always seemed to be "on vacation"—i.e., in a drug rehabilitation center—or asleep in her bedroom.

According to Amy Hochman, Jack's sister, from the outside the Hochmans still looked pretty normal during this time. Occasionally, Pam would stumble or slur a word, and people would start to whisper, but mostly what friends, neighbors, and family—at least the Hochman side of the family—saw in Pam was an attractive, charming, socially poised young woman who was a somewhat erratic mother. "Peter Pan–like" is how Amy describes Pam's parenting then. Like a story-book character, Pam would descend on Romy, shower her with gifts, attention, and love for four or five weeks, then abruptly withdraw.

Pam describes her parenting much more harshly than Amy. She can remember times when baby Romy went a day without a diaper change and times when toddler Romy would find her passed out on the living room couch. Once, Pam brought eighteen-month-old Romy to a fingerprinting session at the Laurel Police Department.

One of the most puzzling things about the Hochman story is why Jack, an earnest, middle-class Amherst graduate, tolerated Pam's drug taking for so long. Jack offers two explanations. One, he was worn down—beaten down—by Pam. And two, after a while, her behavior, the drugs, the upside-down world the Hochmans lived in, began to seem normal to him.

In 1987, a few months after the Hochmans moved to Smithtown, Jack opened the first of the Hochmans' five Long Island TCBY franchises. Pictures of Romy taken after the move to Smithtown show a tall, thin child with short, very blond hair and a long jaw that ends in a prominent chin. Everyone remembers that the Smithtown Romy liked the guitar, *MTV*, lobster, sushi, and basketball, and hated rap music, math, and a classmate named Michelle Epstein. Friends and relatives also remember that during the Hochmans' early years in Smithtown, Romy rarely smiled. Most people blamed this on the family situation, but no one knew for sure; Romy confided in people as infrequently as she smiled.

In 1989, when she was nine, Romy's first Smithtown life came to an end.

One night in early June, she opened the front door and found two men standing on the porch. One of the men flashed a Suffolk County police badge.

"Does Pamela Hochman live here?" he asked.

Romy said her mother was not home now.

The detective looked at his partner, then back at Romy.

"Well, tell her that she's wanted for resisting arrest and attempting to obtain prescription drugs with an illegal prescription."

A month later, Jack sued for divorce and custody of Romy.

After the Hochmans' marriage ended, Romy's life began to assume a regularity and orderliness it had lacked before. She lived in Smithtown with her father, saw her mother, who had moved to Los Angeles, two or three times a year, developed a small circle of friends, and relied on a cast of surrogate mothers—principally Amy and Jack's mother, Eileen—for female role models. Everyone, including Romy, assumed that this new life would last at least until college.

But when she stepped out of the car on that blustery March Sunday in 1994, this second Smithtown life ended, too. As soon as Romy's foot touched the ground, she felt a sharp, daggerlike pain in the lower quadrant of her knee.

"Oww, oww." She slumped against the car and began to massage the knee.

A muscle cramp, Jack thought. Romy had been sitting in the car with her right leg tucked up under her since the McDonald's stop. "Can you walk?" he asked.

Romy put her right leg on the ground again and took a step. This time the pain was not as intense.

"Yeah. I think so," she replied.

"Probably a charley horse," Jack said. "See if you can walk it out."

Romy hobbled around in front of the car for a minute or two. "It feels better now," she said.

The next day Romy woke up to a dull ache where the pain had been. Three days later the ache vanished. But the following week at Theresa Lagado's house, the knee issued another angry warning. While she was running into Theresa's kitchen, Romy's right leg suddenly gave way under her. The next thing she knew, she was lying on the floor looking up at Theresa.

"You okay?" Theresa asked.

Romy said yes, but getting up, she felt a sharp pain in her right knee. However, she did not associate this new pain with the old pain in the car; two weeks is an eternity to a fourteen-year-old.

For the next few weeks the pain kept its own erratic schedule. It would visit for a day, disappear for two or three days, then reappear. But sometime around the middle of May, Romy's discomfort became chronic. It was almost as if the pain had decided to befriend her. Swelling also developed. Nothing dramatic, but standing in front of the mirror with her legs together, Romy could see a slight difference between her left and right knees.

However, Dr. James Little,* Romy's pediatrician, failed to see anything unusual.

"The right and left knee look the same to me," he told Romy when he examined her the Friday before Memorial Day weekend. Dr. Little also saw nothing out of the ordinary in her X ray. He told Jack that the knee in the X ray looked perfectly healthy.

*Pseudonym

Jack gazed at the black-and-white photo in the pediatrician's hand. The whitish hue around the proximal tibia reminded him of the aura night snow gives off.

Dr. Little said he would reexamine the knee in three weeks. In the meantime, Romy's blood tests might reveal something.

"The blood test came back positive for rheumatoid arthritis," Dr. Little said ten days later. The pain was too intense to wait three weeks; Jack had brought Romy back early. Dr. Little explained that rheumatoid arthritis was sort of a "junior arthritis"; it could easily explain the discomfort in the knee. Romy should see a specialist, a rheumatologist, the pediatrician said.

"Panatella of the condrum," the rheumatologist declared, a week later.

Romy was confused. "What about junior arthritis?"

The rheumatologist, Leon Minelli,* shook his head. "A false-positive result. Panatella of the condrum," he said again.

"Pantelina . . ." Romy tried to pronounce the name of her new illness but couldn't. "Panatella of the condrum." This time Romy pronounced the name correctly. "What is it?"

"Growing pains," Dr. Minelli explained. Romy was experiencing discomfort because the panatella bone, which is located in the front section of the knee, was growing faster than the bones adjacent to it. This had the effect of pushing the kneecap sideways. Dr. Minelli illustrated the point by pushing his palm sideways across his chest. The rheumatologist was so sure of his diagnosis, he clung to it through four different sets of blood tests. However, when the last two tests came back positive for Lyme disease, he prescribed a regimen of antibiotics.

"Will the drugs make the pain go away?" asked Romy, who now needed three Advils to fall asleep at night.

"Yes, as soon as the antibiotics get the Lyme disease under control," Dr. Minelli said.

*Pseudonym

But the pain did not go away. In early July it became so bad, it began to wake Romy at night. The first time this happened she was startled to find herself lying on a strange couch in a strange apartment. Then she remembered: she was in Los Angeles. The apartment belonged to her mother, Pam, whom she was visiting for the month of July, and she was sleeping on the couch because her mother's boyfriend was staying over. For a moment, Romy focused on the pain in her knee; she tried to define its character. While it often seemed to encompass the whole leg, if you concentrated hard, as Romy was doing now, you realized that the pain only extended below the knee to the top of the calf muscle and above it to the bottom of the quadriceps. That was the pain's entire domain, its kingdom. The discomfort in the rest of the leg was simply spillover from this area. Dr. Minelli called it "referred pain."

Romy reached for the Advil on the coffee table. Then she remembered: Pam had put the bottle in her purse, and the purse was on a chair in the bedroom. Romy got off the couch and half limped into the bedroom.

Bang! The wastebasket next to the nightstand fell over. Romy was glad she had hit it with her good leg. A rustling sound. Someone was waking up. Was it Pam's boyfriend, Richard? Romy liked Richard, but it was the middle of the night; he might think she was in here spying on him and Pam.

"Rom, is that you?"

Pam's voice; Romy felt relieved.

"Yeah, Mom. I'm looking for the Advil."

The light went on.

"Do you want me to get up with you, hon?"

Romy shook her head. "No, go back to sleep. I'll be okay."

Pam was thrilled to have Romy here, though she worried about her daughter's pain. In October 1993, after conquering her drug problems, Pam moved to California with a dream. In a year or two, when her own life was together, she would ask Romy to come and live with her.

Jack says this story is just that, a story, another Pam pipe dream. He says that if what happened had not happened, then pretty, charming, selfish Pam would have stayed in L.A. and done what she had done in Maryland and in Smithtown: tended her own garden, built a new life for herself, and ignored Romy except for a few weekly visits each year. But what happened did happen, and Jack acknowledges that it became a transforming—a redemptive—experience for Pam. "It gave her life again."

"The antibiotics didn't help at all?" Dr. Minelli seemed surprised—or disappointed, Romy could not tell which. It was the end of July now. And the pain, an ache before California, was now a throb. Yesterday, at Kennedy Airport, Romy had practically hobbled off the plane.

Dr. Minelli looked at the knee again. The left side was slightly swollen, but there were no dramatic changes.

"You're still having pain?"

"Worse pain," Romy said.

Dr. Minelli wrote a prescription for a more powerful antibiotic. However, the rheumatologist did not X-ray the knee. Romy had been to see him three times now and he was still using the X ray Dr. Little had taken in May.

"Do you think this new stuff will work?" Romy asked her father on the drive home.

"Sure," Jack said, but Jack was not sure of anything anymore. Lately he had begun to develop a sense of foreboding. One day very soon, he felt, something bad—something truly awful—was going to leap out of the dark and roll right over him and flatten him.

August was a wonderfully happy time for Romy. She was at her favorite place, her grandfather's house on the Delaware shore, with her favorite cousin, Hanan Katz-Lewis, and at least temporarily, part of a family, a real family—the Katz-Lewis family of San Francisco, California. There were Jackie and Howie, their children, Hanan and Yaffee, and their other child, Romy. For a while that August, even the knee went on vacation. Romy had no pain until the new antibiotic ran out in the middle of the month. But then, refreshed from two weeks of Delaware sun, the pain returned in full force.

On August 20, Romy called Jack and asked him to get the prescription refilled.

"Why don't you come home?" Jack asked. "We'll go see Minelli."

"I don't want to come home. I'm having too much fun."

Romy failed to mention that her knee now looked as if it had two kneecaps. A few days earlier, it had suddenly ballooned up.

Jack asked about the pain.

"I only have a little," Romy lied. She wanted to be part of the Katz-Lewis family for a little longer.

Jack hesitated. He didn't want to ruin Romy's vacation. God knows, after all she had been through, she was entitled to a little fun.

"All right," he said. "Stay." He would call Minelli and make an appointment for the week after Labor Day. In the meantime, he would get Romy's prescription refilled.

Romy saw Dr. Minelli again on September 8 and the doctor seemed stunned when he saw how swollen her knee was.

"That's not the same knee I saw a month ago," he told Jack.

"Same knee, same patient," Jack said.

The rheumatologist finally decided to take his own X ray.

When he reappeared in the office, he seemed different: quieter, more sober. He sat down and looked at Jack.

"Your daughter has a tumor on her knee, Mr. Hochman."

Romy made a strange, whimpering sound.

"It's a benign tumor, Romy," Dr. Minelli said quickly.

"You're sure it's benign?" Jack asked.

Dr. Minelli gave Jack the name of an orthopedic surgeon, a Dr. Paul Aaronson.* But he did not answer the question about the tumor, and Jack did not ask it again; he was afraid to. Now he thought he knew the

*Pseudonym

120

name of the awful thing that was going to come out of the dark and roll over him.

September 8, 1994, was also the day a U.S. Air jetliner crashed on approach to Pittsburgh International Airport. In Los Angeles, Pam and her sister, Lisa, were watching a videotape of the crash on TV when the phone rang in the antiques store they owned.

"Hi, Mom."

Pam knew Romy was supposed to be seeing Dr. Minelli today. "What did the doctor say, hon?"

"He says I have a tumor on my knee, but it's benign. Dad thinks they can take care of it outpatient with orthoscopic surgery."

Pam thought Romy's words might make more sense if she repeated them herself. "You have a tumor on the knee and your father thinks they can take care of it outpatient."

"With orthoscopic surgery," Romy said.

Lisa turned around. "Who has a tumor?" On the screen behind her the nose of the plane was disappearing inside a plume of flames.

Pam mouthed the word "Romy," then turned back to the receiver. "Is your father there, hon? I'd like to talk to him for a minute."

Romy said that Jack had gone back to work.

After Romy hung up, Pam called Dr. Minelli's office.

"Hello, this is Pamela Hochman."

Pam was surprised. The secretary recognized her name immediately. "I know Dr. Minelli wants to talk to you, Mrs. Hochman; he's with a patient now. Give me your number. I'll have him call you back as soon as he's free."

As soon as Pam said, "two-one-three," the secretary became distraught. "That's a Los Angeles area code. You're in Los Angeles?"

Pam said yes.

"Oh dear, it must be terrible, being so far away at a time like this."

Pam noticed that her hand had begun to tremble. She thanked the secretary for her concern and said she would like to speak to Dr. Minelli the moment he was free.

The television was replaying the crash video for the umpteenth time. "Too much," Pam said and stood up. She was about to shut off the TV when the phone rang.

Dr. Minelli was direct and to the point. Romy, he said, had a tumor about the size of a peach on her knee. It was located in the proximal tibia in the left center of the knee. "That's a bad position, Mrs. Hochman. If it had been a little higher or a little lower the situation wouldn't be so serious."

Pam said that Romy had described the tumor as benign.

"I know. That's my fault." Dr. Minelli suddenly sounded contrite. "I saw how upset she got when I said 'tumor.' So I told her it was benign. I shouldn't have, but I haven't had much experience with this kind of thing. You know . . . a child . . . cancer."

Pam did not reply immediately. She needed a moment to digest that last word.

"So you're telling me it's definitely malignant."

"There's a small chance it's an inflammation, an infection." But the rheumatologist said he was not optimistic. "Mrs. Hochman . . ."

"Yes," Pam said.

"I've told your husband already. It's important for both of you to know: The knee I saw today . . . it's not the same knee I saw a month ago." When she hung up, Pam wondered why Minelli had to say that now, in this conversation. Couldn't he have waited a day or two before he started trying to cover himself?

CHAPTER TWO

WHACK! THE SCREEN DOOR SLAMMED CLOSED BEHIND PAM; SHE PUT her suitcase down and looked around. Jack's new house was depressing in the gloomy, unlived-in way only a man can make a house depressing. There were clothes over everything and cheap Holiday Inn furniture everywhere; all of it decorated in Brady Bunch yellows and browns. Poor Romy. The Hochmans' old house on Cedar Street had been so wonderful: overhanging maples, a pool, a lovely front lawn, a circular driveway, twelve large rooms, exposures that caught the sun at every hour of the day. But that house was gone now, everything was gone now: The Hochmans' marriage, the TCBY franchises, the silver Mercedes, the racehorse, the jewelry, the high living . . . nothing was left.

Jack described this new house—actually a five-room apartment attached to someone else's house—as a way station. As soon as he identified the next big thing in fast food, he and Romy would be gone. This was his special gift, Jack believed; he had been endowed with the capacity to see a fast-food trend before anyone else, before it even happened. He had gotten into yogurt ahead of everyone else, hadn't he—and what a killing he made there—and into fast-food chicken, too. (ChickenAmerica!, his one failure, Jack insisted, was a management failure.) This morning, on the way out to Smithtown from Kennedy Airport, Jack told Pam that he had seen the future yet again. This time, he said, it was round and had a hole in the middle. Bagels! Bagels, he announced, were going to be the next big thing in fast food.

There was one problem, though. Beatrice Foods, Jack's last employer, was claiming that he let his major medical plan lapse in May when he left the company to open the bagel business. "Technically, I don't have any medical insurance now."

"But you did renew your major medical?" Pam said.

"Sure I did. I converted it to a private policy. The computer screwed up. They'll sort it out eventually."

On the drive in from the airport, Jack and Pam also made a tentative truce. For now, Pam would stay in the guest bedroom at Jack's. Everything else, including how long Pam stayed in New York, would be determined by what the doctors had to say about Romy's knee. Neither of them mentioned that today, September 11, 1994, was—or would have been—their seventeenth wedding anniversary.

Jack and Dr. Minelli had managed to make the tumor sound like an odd type of sports injury, something you could almost get playing soccer or volleyball. But Dr. Paul Aaronson, the orthopedist the Hochmans saw the next day, was a specialist in sports injuries and he said the shadow on Romy's X ray looked like no sports injury he had ever seen. He told Pam and Jack that the shadow was "ominous."

What a terrible word—*ominous*—Romy thought on the drive home; much worse than *tumor*. Benignly ominous, or ominously benign: you could position the two words any way you wanted, you still ended up with an oxymoron; nothing benign can be ominous and nothing ominous can be benign.

"You can see the tumor in the first X ray. Here. I'll show it to you." It was the following Tuesday, and the Hochmans were sitting in a conference room at the Hospital for Joint Diseases. At Dr. Aaronson's request, Dr. Richard Malloy,* a surgeon there, had agreed to see Romy on two days' notice. Dr. Malloy removed an X ray from a manila folder and stepped in front of an illuminated wall panel. "Here." Dr. Malloy pinned the X ray to the panel. "This is the X ray Dr. Little took in May.

"See? The mass is right there." Dr. Malloy drew a circle around a shadowy formation in the middle of the photo. The area inside the blue line was about the size of an apricot. "There, can you see it?" Dr. Malloy gave the circle a sharp rap with his knuckle.

Jack said he was confused. How could Dr. Little miss a tumor that large?

The surgeon shrugged. "Dr. Little is a pediatrician." Dr. Minelli's failure to take his own X ray until September was passed over in silence. "Now, let me show you the X ray I took this morning." Dr. Malloy picked up another photo from the table and clipped it to the panel. The circle he drew on this photo was notably larger—truly the size of a peach. There was a good chance the mass inside the circle was a tumor, the surgeon said. The mass looked "ominous"—there was that word again. However, Dr. Malloy did not close the door to hope. An X ray was never conclusive; the mass could still turn out to be an infection. "I don't want anyone to panic yet." Dr. Malloy said he wanted his associate, Dr. Donald Pearlman,* to examine the knee.

The next morning, Dr. Pearlman gave the lump a new name, a name even harder to pronounce than "panatella of the condrum." A definitive diagnosis would require a biopsy, Dr. Pearlman cautioned, but there was a better than 50 percent chance the mass on Romy's knee was a form of cancer known as osteosarcoma (OS).

A few minutes later, Pam was standing in front of the hospital, having a cigarette, when Romy walked out of the revolving doors without the crutches Dr. Minelli had prescribed for her. "You know Minelli doesn't want you stressing the knee," Pam said.

"I don't care what Minelli says," Romy yelled. Then she half ran,

*Pseudonym

half hobbled into the street. She was almost on the other side when Jack came out of the hospital. Pam grabbed the crutches from him and ran after Romy. But the light had changed; Pam halted at the curb and looked across Second Avenue.

A group of construction workers were standing in a knot about half a block south on the opposite side of the street. Romy suddenly darted out from behind one of them. A moment later she disappeared into a group of women farther down the block. She was heading south. Pam began walking south on her side of the street. The light at the corner of Seventeenth Street turned red; Pam darted across the avenue. "You know you're not supposed to walk on that knee!" she said when she caught up with Romy in front of a Baskin-Robbins near Sixteenth Street.

"I don't care. It doesn't matter." Romy began to walk again.

"Here. Take them." Pam held out the crutches.

"It doesn't matter!" Romy continued walking.

"What do you mean, it doesn't matter. Of course it matters." Pam grabbed Romy by the shoulder and spun her around. "What do you mean it doesn't matter, young lady?"

"I have cancer. I'm going to die anyway. So what difference does it make?"

Pam dropped the crutches, threw her arms around Romy and hugged her.

On the way back to Smithtown that afternoon, Jack told Pam that Dr. Pearlman would do a knee biopsy the following Tuesday. But he did not tell her that Pearlman was demanding to be paid in advance. "I'm sorry, Mr. Hochman," the surgeon had said the day before, "but that's office policy when the patient doesn't have insurance."

That night, Jack called his father. George Hochman had some money put away for his retirement; he told Jack he could have it to pay for Romy's surgery.

.   .   .

A week later, Pam was standing at a nurses' station at the Hospital for Joint Diseases when a gurney emerged from a side corridor; two Jamaican orderlies were pushing it toward the post-op recovery room. Romy was lying on top, sweaty and unconscious.

"They gave her a general anesthetic," a nurse at the station said. "She won't wake up for another ten minutes." Pam nodded and walked into the recovery room; the orderlies were transferring Romy from the gurney to a bed. After they left, Pam walked over to the bed. Romy began to mumble, then shook her head. The plastic breathing device in her nostrils fell out.

Pam bent down and refastened the device.

Look at this. Here I am, living my life in California and look at what has happened to my daughter. What has my life been?

A nurse appeared. She checked Romy's IV tubing. Pam noticed that a blackish-yellow bruise was beginning to form on the skin around the IV needle.

Am I responsible for this? Is this how God is punishing me? Giving my daughter cancer?

Later, a social worker told Pam that guilt is a common parental reaction to a child's cancer. Parents convince themselves that what happened would not have happened if only things had been done differently: if only the child had not been weaned so early, or not been allowed to eat so much junk food or play in a garden sprayed with insecticides.

Pam did not find the social worker's words comforting.

"I'll give Pearlman another hour," Jack said when he phoned from the office at two-thirty. "Then I'm going to call him. I'll explode if I have to go through the weekend without knowing."

"We'll all explode," Pam said. She was sitting on the bed in the guest room of Jack's house.

Dr. Pearlman had promised to call with the biopsy results the previous day, Thursday, the twenty-seventh; it was now Friday afternoon.

Jack asked where Romy was.

"Downstairs on the couch," Pam said. "Theresa's coming over after school."

For the last few days, Romy had spent almost every waking hour with Theresa and her other best friend Clarissa. She refused to talk about her knee or the visits to the doctors and the hospital—at least to her parents.

"How are you doing?" Pam asked.

"Me?" Jack said. "I'm okay."

The night of the biopsy, Jack had broken down at the kitchen table.

"If you don't hear anything by three," Pam said, "call Pearlman."

Forty-five minutes later, the phone in the guest bedroom rang again. "The biopsy was positive," Jack said. "It's bone cancer."

"Bone cancer?" Osteosarcoma was a soft, squishy word, but bone cancer—bone cancer sounded like the crack of a gunshot, hard and sharp and evil. Pam could tell: she was going to have to say the two words over and over again before she could really believe them.

Romy had an appointment with Dr. Aaron Rausen at five-thirty. Rausen was a pediatric oncologist at New York University Medical Center. "According to Pearlman, he's one of the top cancer specialists in the city."

"He's a big deal, Rausen?" Pam wanted to be told that Rausen was the greatest cancer doctor in the world.

"According to Pearlman, he's *the* expert on osteosarcoma." Romy should pack an overnight bag, Jack said. Pearlman thought Rausen would admit her for the night.

A few minutes before five, Jack dropped Pam and Romy off in front of Dr. Rausen's office, then went to look for a parking space. Immediately inside the lobby there was a directory. Pam stopped and examined it. U, V, R . . . Rogers, Rothstein. Ah, there it was: Rausen, Aaron, eighth floor. A pang of disappointment—Rausen's name was the same size as the other doctors' names. Pam wanted it to be in large neon letters that said DR. AARON RAUSEN, WORLD'S GREATEST CANCER DOCTOR.

She pressed the elevator button and turned around. Romy was standing under a bank of television monitors at the other end of the lobby; the screens above her head all contained the same image: people stepping in and out of elevators.

The elevator doors opened.

"Rom, hon."

Romy's reaction to the biopsy report had been muted. She cried, of course, but not angry, why-did-this-happen-to-me tears. Romy, Pam thought, half regarded the OS as preordained; half believed, maybe more than half believed, that it was Romy Hochman's destiny to have bad things happen to her, the way other girls believed it was their destiny to be pretty or popular or smart. Romy only asked one question about the biopsy. What did osteosarcoma mean? Pam had told her, bone cancer.

The elevator doors opened onto a bright, cheerful waiting room decorated with crayon drawings and photographs of young children. Cancer makes you a connoisseur of luck, and Pam, already an apprentice connoisseur, saw a tiny sliver of luck in the timing of Romy's appointment. At three, the waiting room would have been full of small bald heads, but it was after five and there was only one other child here now. He was sitting on the couch with his mother; blessedly, he had a full head of hair.

Pam walked over to the reception desk; her daughter, Romy Hochman, had an appointment with Dr. Rausen at five-thirty, she said. The receptionist asked her to take a seat, then picked up the phone.

A few minutes later, a bald man in his early sixties stopped at the counter, whispered something to the receptionist, then turned around and walked over to Pam and Romy. "I'm Dr. Rausen," he said. "You must be the Hochmans."

Pam nodded. She liked Dr. Rausen's face immediately. It was round and warm and intelligent-looking. She could tell just by looking at him that he knew more about cancer, about osteosarcoma, than anyone else in New York, than anyone else in America.

"Is your husband here, Mrs. Hochman?"

"He's parking the car."

Dr. Rausen said he had one last patient to see. After that, the Hochmans could have all the time they needed.

"A nice Jewish grandfather," Pam said to Romy, after Dr. Rausen left. "Cuddly."

"Uh-huh," Romy replied. But she was not as taken by Dr. Rausen as her mother. He looked like a businessman to her. A very busy businessman. The smile, the greeting, everything about him had seemed perfunctory and rushed.

A cancer interview is unlike anything else in medicine. Every unspoken thought, every unspoken fear is brought out, examined, and assigned a number. The patient learns the percentage of people who have her type of cancer, her size tumor, her stage of disease, what percentage live and die. She learns what percentage of people develop leukemia from her chemotherapy regimen and what percentage develop heart disease. Life and death are rounded out to the last decimal point.

Two numbers in particular dominated Romy's cancer interview—sixty and sixty-five. Dr. Rausen said the cure rate for adolescent osteosarcoma was 60 percent, except in those cases in which it was 65 percent. Pam was puzzled by this. A week ago, Dr. Pearlman quoted an 80 percent cure rate. How could the cure rate drop fifteen, twenty points in a week? On the news tonight would Peter Jennings report that the breast cancer cure rates had jumped twenty points today, but due to unseasonably cold weather in the Northeast, osteosarcoma was down fifteen points? The drop seemed inexplicable. Pam raised her hand. It was a little girl thing to do, she knew. But there was also a formality, a gravity, about this interview.

"You have a question, Mrs. Hochman?"

Dr. Rausen was seated opposite Pam at the end of a long conference table. Jack, who had joined them, and Romy were seated in between. The room around the table was small, airless, and windowless. It felt claustrophobic.

Pam said yes. "About the cure rates . . ."

"I'll answer questions at the end, Mrs. Hochman. "Dr. Pearlman has already told you that your daughter has osteosarcoma?""

Jack and Pam nodded.

"Osteosarcoma, as you know, is a form of bone cancer," Dr. Rausen said. Then he reeled off the disease's vital statistics: 400 to 600 new cases a year; age group most vulnerable: twelve to eighteen; disease begins in a distal limb like the leg or the arm and usually metastasizes to the lung. Although osteosarcoma's cause is unknown, some evidence suggests it may be triggered by the adolescent growth spurt.

Undoubtedly, Dr. Rausen had given this speech dozens of times before. But Pam still wished he could put a little feeling into it. He sounded as if he were reading from the telephone book.

Romy's prospects of recovery were good, he continued. But treatment for OS was not without risk. Dr. Rausen cleared his throat and began to read from the telephone book again.

Romy would probably never be able to have children.

Romy would lose her hair.

Romy would be at higher risk of developing breast cancer and leukemia as an adult.

Romy would be at higher risk of developing heart disease.

Pam glanced over at Romy, who looked as if she were in a trance.

Romy could develop bladder disease.

Romy could develop liver disease.

Romy could develop lung disease.

Romy could develop skin disease.

But Romy would probably get to keep her leg.

Suddenly, Romy looked wide awake again.

"We didn't know Romy was in danger of losing her leg," Jack said.

"It used to happen all the time; it's fairly rare now, though."

Pam asked about the cure rates again. She was too overwhelmed to process anything else.

Dr. Rausen explained that the 80 percent cure rate was based on one recent study. Most reports showed cure rates of between 60 and 65 percent. But this might change soon. He said a new OS treatment was in clinical trial at NYU. "I think Romy would be a good candidate."

Pam and Jack exchanged glances again.

"It can only benefit her," Dr. Rausen said. "Children who participate in cancer trials have an overall survival rate of 75 percent, compared to a 50 percent survival rate for kids who are treated individually."

Jack said he liked the idea of new treatment.

Pam was less enthusiastic. New meant untried and untested, but, she reasoned, it also meant state-of-the-art. "All right," she said.

"Good. I'll put Romy's name on the trial list." Dr. Rausen looked down at his watch. "Six-thirty. If we hurry, we can still get her into surgery."

Dr. Pearlman had not said anything about surgery tonight.

"What kind of surgery?" Jack asked.

"The Broviac." Dr. Rausen explained that chemotherapy was administered into the body via a metal catheter called a Broviac; it had to be implanted surgically into the chest. The sooner Romy had a Broviac, the sooner treatment could start.

Later, Romy would say that the only thing she remembers about this interview was Dr. Rausen's announcement at the end about the surgery, that and the feeling she had when she left the room. At that moment, she says, she hated Aaron Rausen more than she had ever hated anyone in her entire life.

CHAPTER THREE

MODERN CHEMOTHERAPY IS A HEROIC TREATMENT, SO IT IS APPROPRI-
ate that it began in a heroic circumstance: a wartime bombing raid.

One day in the summer of 1943, German planes attacked the Italian port city of Bari and sank several Allied ships, among them an
American tanker with a top secret cargo: mustard gas.

The crew of the tanker knew nothing about the secret cargo. But
within a few days, the sailors did know that the yellow slime they dived
into after the raid contained something unhealthy. Everyone in the crew
was violently ill. The Army medical officer in Bari quickly identified the
source of the illness. The mustard gas had (temporarily) destroyed the
men's white blood cells, producing the classic symptoms of aplastic
anemia: high fever, vomiting, whole-body rashes. There the matter
might have rested, except for a quirk of military bureaucracy. Since the
incident involved mustard gas, the medical officer's report was for-
warded to Colonel C. P. Rhodes in the Army's Department of Chemical
Warfare.

The sailors' symptoms intrigued Colonel Rhodes, who in civilian life was an oncologist. Two particularly deadly cancers, leukemia and lymphoma, were both characterized by out-of-control white blood cell production; a substance capable of shutting down this production might have value as an anticancer drug. Colonel Rhodes mentioned the medical officer's findings about mustard gas to a former colleague, Yale pharmacologist Albert Gilman. Six months later, a lymphoma patient at Yale–New Haven Hospital received the world's first chemotherapeutic agent, mustard nitrate, an analog of mustard gas.

The modern era of chemotherapy had begun.

In 1946, cancer patient Babe Ruth brought the new treatment to public attention when he was treated with a variant of mustard nitrate at Mount Sinai Hospital in New York. However, it was a physician, Dr. Sidney Farber of Boston Children's Hospital, who made chemotherapy a household word. In 1947, Dr. Farber actually produced remissions in a few children with leukemia, a disease unremittingly fatal in the late 1940s. According to Dr. Ezra Greenspan, professor emeritus of medicine at Mount Sinai Medical School, after Farber's success everyone in oncology was sure: the cure for cancer was at hand.

A half century later, though, the overall survival rate for adult cancer, 60 percent, is not dramatically better than it was in the 1950s. But pediatric oncology has come close to attaining the kind of success Dr. Greenspan and his colleagues dreamed of. Today, 75 percent of children with cancer are saved.

Luck—never to be underestimated in medicine—has had something to do with this success. The early chemotherapeutic agents all turned out to work better against childhood cancers, like leukemia and the sarcomas (cancers of the connective tissue, such as muscle and bone), than against adult carcinomas—cancers of the lining cells of the internal organs (such as the liver or lung), glands (such as the breast or prostate), and of the skin.

Pediatric oncologists can also deploy more drugs against pediatric cancers; with dosages adjusted for body weight, a child can tolerate significantly higher quantities of chemotherapy than an adult.

A third reason for the high cure rate in childhood cancer is an unusually large and sophisticated clinical trials network. Every year, 80 percent of the children diagnosed with cancer are triaged into a study; this allows pediatric oncology to test and disseminate new therapies far more quickly than adult oncology, where only 2 to 3 percent of patients participate in clinical trials. Indeed, many regimens used against adult cancers were first tested on children.

Osteosarcoma, however, is an exception to this rule. Chemotherapy, a standard adult treatment since the mid-1960s, did not become a standard treatment against OS until the mid-1980s, when the Multi-Institutional Osteosarcoma Study (MIOS), one of the most controversial studies ever conducted, established chemo as the treatment of choice against osteosarcoma.

Until MIOS, osteosarcoma was a disease devoid of hope. No one knew what caused it or how to treat it. However, the natural history of OS had been well known for over a hundred years.

Osteosarcoma, almost exclusively a disease of early adolescence, strikes children in the twelve-to-eighteen age group. Because the human body grows fastest in these years, many oncologists believe that rapid growth somehow acts as a trigger in OS; many statistics support this view. Girls, who shoot up earlier than boys, usually get OS earlier; and fast-growing tall children have higher rates of the disease than slow-growing short youngsters.

Current thinking explains the relationship between rapid growth and OS this way: Somehow, the abrupt increase in bone cell production during early adolescence knocks out p53, one of the "regulator" genes responsible for keeping rapid cell growth under control. We know that a knocked-out regulator gene leads to a pediatric eye cancer called retinoblastoma (RB). When the RB regulator gene is "hit," retinal cell production swings out of control and takes on a wild, cancerlike pattern.

Many oncologists believe that something similar happens to bone cell production when the p53 gene is hit.

An alternate theory holds that osteosarcoma is somehow triggered by an injury, since the disease frequently occurs in the knees, hips, and shoulders—common areas of childhood injury.

In OS, the average duration between the appearance of symptoms and diagnosis is only three months, although Dr. Michael Link of Stanford University says a six-month history like Romy's is not uncommon. Also typical is the way OS announced itself to Romy—as sharp jabbing pain. On occasion, though, the presenting symptoms are more dramatic. One of Dr. Rausen's patients, a sixteen-year-old girl, was entirely asymptomatic until she leaned against a wall one day. The girl felt a sudden, sharp, hot pain in her shoulder, then heard a cracking sound. Her shoulder bone, eaten through with cancer, had just broken in two.

Osteosarcoma's most unnerving characteristic is its metastatic capacity. Like other cancer cells, malignant bone cells retain a rudimentary ability to perform the task they were designed for. Thus, as the disease spreads, small bone-building calcium deposits begin to appear in other parts of the body, particularly in the lung. As many as 80 percent of OS patients are thought to have lung metastases at the time of diagnosis.

Children like Romy do not usually die from bone tumors; they die from great galloping lung tumors—tumors that waste the trunk and face and produce gasping, old-man breathing in thirteen- and fourteen-year-olds. In many cases of OS, the official cause of death is pulmonary insufficiency. Essentially, the child suffocates to death.

In the 1920s, a famous surgeon closed an OS conference with this cry: "Gentlemen, they die if we operate, they die if we don't operate. This meeting should be concluded with prayers." Thirty years later, prayer remained the only hope for an OS child. In 1950, the survival rate for the disease was 10 percent, and the treatment of choice, as it had been in 1920, was whole-limb amputation. In 1970, the situation was a little better. Twenty percent of OS children survived, and surgery was limited to tumor removal; a postoperative course of radiation often followed. Then something miraculous began to happen.

Over the next ten years, the OS survival rate doubled, then nearly doubled again; in 1980, 55 percent to 65 percent of OS kids survived five years or longer. Most people in pediatric oncology had no doubt about the source of the miracle; it was chemotherapy. Survival rates leaped as soon as agents like Adriamycin and methotrexate were introduced into OS treatment in the early 1970s. There had to be a correlation.

But a minority within the profession disagreed. They believed just as strongly that the claims made on behalf of chemotherapy were exaggerated, and their opinion carried special weight because they were affiliated with very prestigious institutions. In the spring of 1981, a group of Mayo Clinic researchers published an editorial in the *Journal of Clinical Oncology* with the deliberately provocative title, "Adjuvant (Post Operative) Chemotherapy in Osteosarcoma: The Promise That Isn't."

Essentially, the paper argued that chemotherapy's success against OS might be an illusion. The Mayo team noted that the claims for chemo's effectiveness rested on the experience of individual doctors at individual institutions—in other words, it rested on anecdotal evidence or something very much like it. No one had ever actually tested chemo head-on against other OS treatments in a large-scale clinical trial, the traditional and most reliable way to determine a treatment's effectiveness.

Furthermore, the Mayo team noted, other equally plausible explanations could account for the sudden jump in OS survival rates. In the 1970s, new diagnostic equipment made early identification and treatment more common. Also, at the start of the decade, most OS cases were still treated in small community hospitals, while at its end, most were treated at major cancer centers, where more sophisticated care and more experienced medical teams were available.

The Mayo team published a second, even more provocative paper a few years later that compared the OS survival rates for surgery plus radiation against survival rates for surgery plus chemotherapy. Statistically, they were virtually the same: 40 percent versus 44 percent.

The second Mayo paper ended as the first had, with a call for a big-numbers, carefully controlled clinical trial of chemotherapy plus surgery versus surgery plus radiation.

Dr. Michael Link of Stanford University says that the ethics of running such a study nearly drove pediatric oncology to civil war in the early 1980s. Many oncologists thought that the Mayo team's proposal was, at the very least, unreasonable. Chemotherapy saved lives; they had seen it with their own eyes. They were not going to put patients' lives—children's lives—at risk just to satisfy a few skeptics in Minnesota; the Mayo proposal was unconscionable, they argued. But the Mayo team and its supporters argued back that it was unconscionable to subject children to very toxic drugs when it was impossible to say with scientific certainty that the drugs worked.

The National Cancer Institute settled the dispute in 1986 when it ordered a head-on study of chemo versus surgery. Memorial Sloan-Kettering, NYU, and many other leading cancer centers refused to participate in what became known as the Multi-Institutional Osteosarcoma Study. But MIOS's lead investigator, Dr. Link, finally did find several willing institutions, including Stanford and Dana Farber in the United States and Great Ormand Street Hospital and Hammersmith Hospital in Great Britain.

The results of the study vindicated the anti-Mayo group. At the end of the second year, the relapse rate among the non-chemotherapy-treated youngsters was *90* percent; the comparable relapse figure for the youngsters in the chemo group was 26 percent. The MIOS trial was immediately suspended.

The relapsed children were eventually saved with a combination of chemotherapy and surgery. But the study left pediatric oncology deeply, profoundly shaken. Children had suffered and, some oncologists believe, a few had died in order to validate a treatment most people in the profession already knew worked.

To avoid future MIOSs, henceforth, every new OS treatment would have to be thoroughly tested *first* in the traditional three-stage clinical trials system; there could be no exceptions.

This conclusion, which seemed wise and prudent at the time, came very close to destroying Romy's trial, Intergroup 0133, the first study to take osteosarcoma beyond chemotherapy.

CHAPTER FOUR

Normally, on a pleasant early autumn evening, the walk from Dr. Rausen's office on Thirty-fourth Street to the NYU Medical Center only takes five minutes. But on the evening of September 14, 1994, it took Pam and Romy, who was still on crutches, nearly fifteen minutes. Walking to the medical center was Romy's idea. She thought it might be weeks—months—before she was outside again; she wanted one last look at normal life.

The medical center's reception area, a Miami Beach–like structure near the corner of Thirtieth Street and First Avenue, was built on an epic New York scale; two stories high and almost half a football field long. Inside, a man in a blue blazer was standing at a blond wooden counter. There was some sort of garden or court behind him. After she helped Romy through the revolving doors, Pam walked over and asked what floor pediatrics was on.

"Nine," the man said in a Spanish accent. He pointed to a corridor that led to the main building. "The elevators are at the other end."

Romy's room, 957, had a wonderful river view, but the window bed was already taken. It was occupied by a girl of about sixteen, with very fine blond-brown hair and large dark eyes. Romy could tell the girl had been quite pretty once, pretty in the almond-eyed, sultry way eastern European gymnasts often are. But cachexia, a symptom of advanced cancer, had pinched all of the prettiness out of her face. Now she just looked very sick and very angry.

The girl introduced herself as Lotte Kauffman and turned toward the window.

"Lotte's a pretty name," Romy said.

"Thank you." The girl did not turn around.

Romy noticed red sores along the girl's arms; the sores looked like mosquito bites that had scabbed over. Romy also noticed that the girl's left leg was missing.

While Romy was in the bathroom changing, the girl began to cough.

"Do you want some water?" Pam asked.

"Thank you, I have—" The girl began to hack again. The cough, which had begun softly, was now suddenly quite deep. The girl sat up in the bed. The coughing seemed to start in the pit of her stomach and ratchet its way up through the rib cage into her chest and throat. When the coughing spasm passed, the girl said, "Thank you, I have some water here." Somehow, she managed to make the statement sound unfriendly. She took a sip from a glass on the nightstand, then lay back on the pillow and closed her eyes.

The clock on the nightstand beside her said 7:15. Pam could hardly believe it. It was only three hours since Dr. Pearlman had spoken to Jack. She felt as if she had risen from the dead at least twice since then.

"Romy Hochman?" A nurse was standing at the door with a wheelchair.

"She's in the bathroom," Pam said. "I'm her mother."

"Dr. Rausen wants her downstairs for a bone scan."

When Romy came out of the bathroom, she asked about the Broviac implant.

"Lucky you, dear," the nurse replied. "Postponed until tomorrow."

Romy did not feel lucky, but she did feel relieved. From the moment Dr. Rausen said, "If we hurry, we can get her into surgery tonight," all Romy had thought about were needles, and Romy hated needles; they were worse than having a peach-sized tumor on your knee, worse than nine months of chemotherapy, worse than being told you will never have children, worse than having a roommate with no leg, worse than anything.

Only much later, when Pam said yes, she was staying in New York, did Romy stop thinking about needles and fall asleep.

Like most human institutions, the pediatrics ward at NYU has its own set of rituals and customs. Some are mystical and irrational; there is, for example, the black magic of the never-speak rule—speak the name of a discharged child and the child will return to the ward ill. Other rituals are more sober and practical. One exclusive to OS families is the sharing of the cell kill count, which is sort of like comparing SAT scores, except that the comparison involves not math and English scores, but the percentage of bone cancer cells killed by chemotherapy. A 70 percent cell kill means that 30 percent of the cancer cells are still alive, while an 85 percent kill means that only 15 percent of the cells are.

The day after Romy was admitted, she and Pam were introduced to the cell kill ritual by Paul Gertz, the father of another OS patient. Pam never found out who sent Paul or how he knew so much about Romy—and about Lotte, who, it turned out, also had OS. But she half suspected Dr. Rausen had; almost the first thing Paul mentioned when he sat down was the new OS study Romy was entering. Paul said his son Daniel was in it and doing very well. "Daniel has a 93 percent cell kill," Paul said. "Eighty percent of OS kids with cell kills in Daniel's range survive into adulthood."

Paul had a nice face, Pam decided: small twinkly eyes, a slightly beaked nose, and a lopsided grin. And he was wonderful with Romy, kind and gentle and considerate.

Just before he left, he told her, "I know you feel like you just fell off the end of the earth. But you haven't. The next nine months are going to be very hard; you're going to have to be brave. But you have a beatable disease. Daniel has beaten it and you can too."

In the hall, Paul told Pam that he had stored samples of Daniel's sperm in a Connecticut sperm bank before the start of chemo; he did not know if there was a similar procedure for eggs, but if Romy wanted to have children someday, the Hochmans ought to look into it. "You have to start thinking ahead," Paul said.

That afternoon, while a team of surgeons implanted a Broviac between Romy's two small adolescent breasts, Pam found herself thinking about cell kill counts. What about the children who got sixty-six or sixty-eight or seventy-two? she wondered. What was the etiquette when your child scored low? Did you lie about a bad score? Pump it up to an eighty-five or an eighty-eight to make it sound respectable, the way you would a low SAT score? Or did you just leave the room when other parents began talking about cell kills? Later that afternoon Pam found herself wondering about Lotte's cell kill. What had it been? For a moment, Pam had an impulse to call up Lotte's parents and ask.

The next day, Sunday, Romy's second full day as a cancer patient, Aaron Rausen visited the Hochmans. He was dressed exactly as he had been at his office, in a weathered gray suit. But Pam noticed something new about him this morning: his walk. Dr. Rausen had a Jimmy Cagney walk: quick, fluid, masculine, but also dainty. It was surprising to see in a portly sixty-year-old doctor.

"Good day to you, Mrs. Hochman." Dr. Rausen bowed his head slightly in Pam's direction.

Pam smiled and said hello. She liked Dr. Rausen's old-fashioned formality. It bespoke a solidity, a certain kind of paternalism that made her feel taken care of. None of the younger doctors she had met in the last four weeks, the eager, friendly, clueless baby boomers who called her Pam, had made her feel that way.

Dr. Rausen bent down and examined the chart at the foot of Romy's bed. Romy watched him warily. Her opinion of Dr. Rausen had not changed either. She still found him distracted and oblivious, still resented the way he talked about her, as if she were an object, a car with a broken carburetor, still hated him for telling her she had cancer.

"And you?" Dr. Rausen said, looking up suddenly. "How are you today, young lady?"

"Fine."

"How's the Broviac?"

"Fine."

"Any discomfort?"

"No."

Dr. Rausen put Romy's chart down on a table and said he had Romy's assignment in Intergroup Trial 0133.

Pam sat up.

The previous Friday, Dr. Rausen had been very enthusiastic about the study. He told the Hochmans that one of the two new drugs in 0133, MTP, was designed to prevent lung metastases, the leading cause of death in osteosarcoma. He also said the four-armed structure of the trial gave Romy a 75 percent chance of receiving at least one new drug, either MTP or the other new agent, Ifosfamide, and a one-in-four chance of receiving both. Pretty good odds for a clinical trial—though, Dr. Rausen was careful to emphasize, odds he had no personal control over.

The study was set up like a telemarketing service, he had said at the meeting. He called an 800 number in Arcadia, California, gave Romy's name and hospital to a telephone operator and the operator gave him an arm assignment. Romy would either be Arm A, which was MTP plus three standard chemotherapy agents; Arm B, Ifosfamide plus the same three traditional agents; Arm C, MTP *and* Ifosfamide plus the three agents; or Arm D, the control group, which got the three standard chemotherapeutic agents alone.

Pam did not remember the letter designations, so when Dr. Rausen said Romy was in Arm D, her initial reaction was confusion.

"D? D is good?" she asked.

Dr. Rausen nodded. D was good. The three trial drugs in the arm—high-dose methotrexate, cisplatin, and Adriamycin—had a wonderful track record.

Romy looked up from the Sunday paper and asked how many of the drugs in D were new. This was the first time she had shown any interest in the conversation.

D was the standard therapy arm of the study, Dr. Rausen said. It had no new drugs. Romy was in the control group.

Suddenly, D did not sound so good to Pam.

"Mrs. Hochman," Dr. Rausen said, "methotrexate, cisplatin, and Adriamycin have cured thousands of children. Arm D is a proven treatment."

"I shouldn't worry, then? I shouldn't feel deprived?"

Dr. Rausen shook his head. Pam was amazed: The two new drugs had already ceased to exist for Dr. Rausen. Poof! Just like that, they were out of his head. Maybe this was a message, Pam thought. Maybe Dr. Rausen was saying, "Mrs. Hochman, unless you want to drive yourself crazy, forget you ever heard of MTP and Ifosfamide."

Later, when they were alone, Pam asked Romy how she felt about her study assignment.

Romy smiled and said, "Relieved." According to the trial protocol, D had the shortest chemotherapy schedule.

Pam's disappointment evaporated that night when she read the protocol for 0133. The brew of flulike symptoms MTP produced—fever, chills, malaise, body aches, and headaches—sounded minor, especially for an anticancer agent. But the risks associated with Ifosfamide, the other new test drug, were terrifying: kidney damage, liver damage, bone marrow depression, confusion, sleeplessness, coma, seizure, decreased sperm count—Pam thought of poor Daniel Gertz when she read that—and acute myelogenous leukemia.

Arm D, she decided, was not such a bad assignment after all.

Pam sat up and adjusted the reading light. Until she moved into Ronald McDonald House at the end of the month, home would be a cot next to Romy's bed.

This morning, when she told Jack about the move, Pam also told him something else, something she had been thinking about ever since returning to New York. "I want to be Romy's mother again," she said over breakfast in the cafeteria. "Romy needs me now."

Jack put down his coffee and looked at her warily. "You mean, you want me to step aside, Pam; you want to be the primary parent now." That was an oddly clinical term to use, Pam thought, "primary parent."

"I want to do this for Romy . . ." she said. "I want to do it for me, Jack."

Jack took another sip of his coffee; when he looked at Pam again, his gaze was softer. "A child needs a mother," he said.

Pam looked down at the protocol. The page was open to high-dose methotrexate, the first of the three drugs Romy would receive in Arm D.

According to the protocol, serious brain damage was an "extremely unusual" side effect of the agent. But bone marrow depression, mouth sores, nausea, vomiting, diarrhea, and decreased liver function were all fairly common.

In addition to nausea, vomiting, and diarrhea, the side effects associated with cisplatin included hearing loss, decreased kidney function, and cancer. According to the protocol, one in every 50 to 800 patients treated with cisplatin developed leukemia.

Adriamycin (doxorubicin), like its two cousins, caused nausea, vomiting, diarrhea, bone marrow depression, and an increased risk of leukemia. But it also posed some hazards of its own: red urine (the protocol noted that this side effect was not dangerous), hair loss, burning or irritation of the tissue, and heart damage, including heartbeat irregularities and heart failure.

There was an informed consent form attached to the protocol. Pam opened the form to page two. Halfway down the page there was a guardian's statement:

"I have read the description of the clinical research study. . . . I understand enough about the purpose, methods, risks, and benefits of the study to judge that I want the patient to take part in it."

Pam looked over at Romy, who was already asleep. Lotte was still looking out the window, though there was nothing to look at but night and a few twinkling lights on the Queens side of the East River.

Pam opened her purse and took out a pen.

On Tuesday, October 2, 1994, Romy's first chemotherapy session was administered in the pediatric ICU; this was an extraordinary precaution. Usually chemo is administered in the patient's room. But Romy was subject to premature ventricular beats (PVC), a form of irregular heartbeat. The combination of PVCs and Adriamycin, a cardiotoxic drug, could produce flatline, or cardiac arrest; Romy's heart rate could shoot up to 250 beats a minute, then stop cold. If flatline occurred, the ICU was the safest place to be.

Romy says that she began to feel nauseated about an hour after she was attached to the cisplatin drip. But she does not remember when she actually started vomiting. Jack and Pam do. Three hours into the treatment, Romy suddenly sat upright and said, "I feel sick," and ejected a stream of yellow-green fluid across the bed. After all the food in her stomach was ejected, Romy vomited her body fluids. Then she just retched.

The nausea and vomiting continued through the first day and night; finally, around ten on the second morning, Romy fell asleep. A few minutes later, Pam heard shouting outside the ICU. *Bang!* The doors flew open; half a dozen men and women burst into the unit at a half run. "Twelve CCs of penicillin!" one demanded. "Kidney failure! He's in kidney failure!" barked another. For a second, Pam half thought the ICU was under terrorist attack. She glanced over at Romy—still asleep, thank God—then back at the staff, who were hustling a gurney with a sweaty, reddish-pink ball on top into the ICU. The ball was a naked child, a boy of about four or five. He was the most grotesquely swollen thing Pam had ever seen. His arms, legs, eyelids—everything about him—was larger and fatter than it should have been, fatter than his little-boy body could sustain. Pam was certain the child was going to explode, burst wide open, any second.

A woman in a hip-length black leather jacket was standing behind the boy. She was about thirty, with dark hair and a gaunt, high-cheekboned face. The woman seemed too stricken to move, to do anything but stare at the child on the gurney. Pam wanted to say something, to offer the woman a word of reassurance, but before she had a chance the woman was whisked to the other end of the ICU. A moment later, the gurney and the crowd of medical personnel disappeared behind a drawn curtain. The whole episode had the fluid, unreal quality of a dream, Pam said later. Sixty seconds after the curtain was drawn, the unit was quiet again. Only an occasional *beep beep* punctured the stillness.

Around one o'clock the next morning, Romy suddenly began to toss and turn frantically.

Pam bent forward. "Rom, honey, are you okay?"

"My leg! My leg hurts. *My leg hurts!*"

"What's the matter?" One of the ICU nurses was at the bed now.

Pam wanted to say, "What a stupid question." Instead she said, "My daughter is having pain in her knee. Do you think she could have some morphine?"

"Morphine?" The request surprised the nurse. "We give codeine pills for pain."

Pam pointed out that Romy was too nauseated to keep a pill down.

"We could grind it up for her," the nurse said.

"I don't think that would help."

"Owwww!" Romy bolted upright on the bed. She rocked back and forth; then suddenly the upper part of her body jackknifed down toward her legs. "Aaaaggghhh!"

"I'll get the resident," the nurse said.

Ten minutes later, a morphine line was plugged into Romy's Broviac. Pam, who was not unfamiliar with the drug, had read somewhere that pain counteracts morphine's euphoric effects. Romy's reaction seemed to confirm this.

She sat up in the bed and said in a strange, sleepwalker's voice, "I feel funny; I feel hot all over."

The nurse who had plugged in the morphine line began to laugh. "Trust me, honey, hot is good. Go with the feeling."

"No! No!"

But in the middle of the protest, Romy collapsed back onto the pillow. When she woke up fourteen hours later, she was in her room again, sunlight was streaming through the window, and the pain in her knee was gone.

CHAPTER FIVE

IN THE SUMMER OF 1978, DR. GREGORY MACEWEN ARRIVED IN NEW York City in the midst of a personal crisis. As a boy, Dr. MacEwen had dreamed of becoming a veterinarian; like James Herriot, he would travel from farm to farm in Wellington boots and an Irish walking hat saving sick animals. But now that he actually was a vet, Dr. MacEwen was finding his chosen profession a little boring and more than a little unfulfilling.

For a while, Dr. MacEwen toyed with the idea of becoming a medical doctor. But that would mean more school and more tuition bills. The compromise Dr. MacEwen struck between his head and his heart was canine oncology; he had come to New York to study at the Animal Medical Center, a world leader in the field.

Canine oncology, Dr. MacEwen believed, would still allow him to help sick animals—a continuing priority—but also to do research that could benefit people.

After his residency, Dr. MacEwen spent the next few years at AMC working on anticancer drugs with crossover potential to humans, mostly mixed bacterial agents and biologics, naturally occurring substances that enhance the body's own defenses against disease. In 1981, Dr. MacEwen's interest narrowed to a particular biologic, one that stimulates the immune system to attack cancer cells, muramyl tripeptide phosphatidyl ethanolamine, or MTP. This was one of the new agents being tested in Romy's study and it was potentially the most important new OS drug in a generation.

Dr. MacEwen, now a professor of veterinary medicine at the University of Wisconsin, first came across MTP in a 1981 issue of *Science* magazine. Scanning the contents page, he saw the name of an old teacher, Isaiah Fidler. Curious, Dr. MacEwen turned to the Fidler article; it described the action of muramyl tripeptide phosphatidyl ethanolamine against malignant melanoma (the most deadly form of skin cancer) in a group of laboratory mice.

The article and Dr. Fidler's work on MTP grew out of an observation he had made about macrophage cells in the early 1970s. Macrophages, among the immune system's most ferocious killers, are also big snackers, particularly of liposomes. When it comes to liposomes, a macrophage can never eat just one. This, Dr. Fidler thought, might make a hollow liposome a good package for an anticancer drug; an "enriched" liposome could enhance the normal killing power of the macrophage that gobbled it up; maybe by a factor of three or four.

The experiment reported in *Science* showed that MTP, the drug Dr. Fidler chose to put inside the "enriched" liposome, was very effective in stimulating the mouse immune system to attack cancer cells. In the conclusion of the *Science* paper, Dr. Fidler stated that MTP, effective against mouse cancers, might one day also be effective against many human cancers. Dr. MacEwen agreed. But he thought that the MTP-liposome combination might help him solve a more immediate problem.

Osteosarcoma, which mostly afflicts large-boned breeds like Great Danes and St. Bernards, is the third leading cause of cancer death in dogs. In the early 1980s, amputation remained the primary treatment for canine OS, and it was about as successful as amputation alone had been in humans a generation earlier. Ninety percent of afflicted dogs were dead within a year, usually from lung metastases. The success of chemotherapy in human OS suggested that a pharmaceutical attack might also work against canine OS. But a chemotherapy strategy posed two problems.

One was cost. In 1981, a single treatment of high-dose methotrexate was $1,200; a single treatment of Adriamycin, then new on the market, was $600. You might get an insurance company to pay those prices for a human patient, but, Dr. MacEwen knew, not many dog owners would. The other problem was toxicity. How many people would willingly subject the family pet to hair loss, nausea, vomiting, and diarrhea, particularly for an as yet unproven treatment? Dr. MacEwen thought, not many.

MTP might solve both the money and toxicity problems. It was a biologic, a natural substance, and thus, unlike chemotherapeutic agents, low in toxicity. Also it did not have to be administered in a $600-a-day dose, like methotrexate.

Dr. MacEwen called Dr. Fidler at the National Cancer Institute, which was a cheeky move for an obscure young vet, since, in 1981, Dr. Fidler was already a marquee name in cancer research. But Dr. Fidler took the call anyway and he was glad he did. It turned out that the young vet had something he wanted.

One of the problems with testing a new drug on specially bred mice is that the animals' look-alike genetic engineering produces uniform tumor growth. In the wild, cancers don't grow that way. A naturally occurring malignancy has its own special characteristics, its own unique biological fingerprint.

How well would MTP work against natural cancers?

Dr. Fidler decided that Dr. MacEwen, who had access to OS dogs, would be the perfect person to provide the answer.

The curious history of MTP begins with a curious fact; it is a relatively weak drug. A big tumor like Romy's could easily shake off its effects. But OS is not in need of big treatments; it already has two, in surgery and chemotherapy, which when combined can kill the primary tumor and most of the surrounding disease. Lung metastases, the principal cause of death in OS, develops from the cancer cells left behind.

The dog study Drs. MacEwen and Fidler designed asked a simple question. Could MTP activate the dogs' own immune systems to kill off this small but deadly residue of cancer cells? Dr. MacEwen removed the primary tumor surgically, then put one group of dogs on a two-month regimen of MTP, while the other group received nothing. The results surprised even Dr. MacEwen. On average, MTP dogs survived three times longer than the untreated animals. A few even achieved a kind of canine immortality; they became the first OS dogs ever to live out their natural life spans.

Researchers get interested in a particular disease for a particular reason. OS attracted Dr. MacEwen because it filled a professional and emotional need. Dr. Eugenie Kleinerman, another important figure in the MTP story, was drawn to the disease by a TV movie about a high school track star who died of osteosarcoma. Dr. Kleinerman still doesn't know why the movie affected her so deeply. "I think maybe, subconsciously, I identified with the pediatrician in the film," she says. "It is a terrible thing to stand by helplessly and watch a child die."

A second epiphany led Dr. Kleinerman to MTP. Every cancer treatment has a natural ceiling; even the best, most broad-gauged therapy will not work for everyone. In the early 1980s, while the rest of pediatric oncology was arguing about whether to use chemo, Dr. Kleinerman was already calculating its natural ceiling in OS. She estimated it to be between 60 and 65 percent; when paired with surgery, that's the percentage of children she thought the treatment could save.

Drugs such as Adriamycin and cisplatin would prolong life, but they would not save the remaining 35 to 40 percent of OS kids. To survive, these youngsters would need something else, something capable of killing chemo-resistant cancer cells.

Five years later, the OS survival rate leveled off where Dr. Kleinerman predicted it would, in the 60-to-65-percent range.

Dr. Kleinerman's interest in MTP grew out of a talk she heard Dr. Fidler give one night in 1983. "As I sat in the audience listening, a lightbulb went on over my head," she says. She realized that OS needed a multistep strategy: surgery and chemotherapy to destroy the primary cancer, and MTP to destroy the residue of chemo-resistant cancer cells before they had a chance to metastasize to the lung. "I wanted to get MTP into clinical trials right away," she says.

Dr. Kleinerman, who was also at the National Cancer Institute, contacted Dr. Fidler about her idea and he immediately invited her to do an in vitro safety study on MTP, which is the first hurdle in testing every new agent.

The reason chemotherapy causes nausea, vomiting, and baldness (among other things) is that it kills all kinds of fast-breeding cells, including hair and stomach cells, which divide nearly as rapidly as cancer cells. Was MTP also an indiscriminate killer? To answer this question, Dr. Kleinerman put a group of healthy cells and cancerous cells into a test tube and added a small amount of MTP. A few hours later, the healthy cells were still alive, the cancer cells dead.

But it took ten to twenty "MTP-enhanced" macrophage cells to kill a single cancer cell, which begged the question: Is raw killing power, the traditional way of evaluating a cancer drug's effectiveness, the best and only way?

Generally, the higher a given cancer's cure rate, the harder the climb up cure mountain becomes. The last third of the climb is always the hardest because the last third of the climb is made up of patients who, through some biological quirk, resist treatments that work for everyone else.

In many ways, the controversy about MTP is also a controversy about how to get to the top of cure mountain. MTP's proponents believe that for the third of kids who live near the top of the mountain, the best measure of a new drug's effectiveness is its ability to destroy the small residue of cancer cells left undestroyed by chemotherapy. MTP's opponents believe that the last third of the mountain should be climbed the way the first two-thirds were—with big, toxic drugs that can Roto-Rooter millions of cancer cells into oblivion.

From the beginning, Dr. Kleinerman knew that the relatively low killing power of MTP would generate opposition, particularly from chemo traditionalists. But she never dreamed that the opposition would be as intense as it turned out to be.

The first problem arose immediately after the end of MTP's initial human study, a phase one clinical trial, which is the first of the three human studies the Food and Drug Administration requires a new treatment to pass. Phase one trials are designed to determine the safest and most effective dose of a new drug, and in the case of cancer drugs, a half century of experience has shown that the best dose to give is the maximum tolerated dose, i.e., the largest amount of drug the patient can tolerate without becoming seriously ill or dying. But the results of the phase one Dr. Kleinerman did on MTP indicated that it actually worked better at less than half its maximum tolerated dose.

MTP flat out failed its phase two trial. A phase two is designed to take a second look at a new drug's safety and a first look at its effectiveness, and in cancer, the chief measure of effectiveness is a drug's ability to visibly shrink a tumor. MTP, a mop-up drug, could not meet the benchmark. By all rights, it should have died in phase two, and it would have, except for one thing—it worked.

After some dosage adjustments, the drug doubled the survival rates among relapsed patients, the most common subjects in phase two trials and also the hardest patients to treat.

Impressed by MTP's performance, in 1989, the Pediatric Oncology Group (POG) invited Dr. Kleinerman to make a case for using the drug in untreated OS patients. The invitation represented *the* big chance for MTP. Only POG, a research consortium of large cancer institutions, or its counterpart, the Children's Cancer Group (through their member institutions), could supply the 400 to 500 patients necessary to do a big, complex phase three, the final step in the drug approval process.

But Dr. Kleinerman knew that MTP would not be an easy sell. The first treatment almost always represents a cancer patient's best chance at a cure. Dr. Kleinerman would have to convince POG that it was justifiable to use that chance on a drug that could not visibly shrink a tumor.

The moral proposition she presented to the consortium was very straightforward: The potential benefit of saving the 35 to 40 percent of OS kids with a residue of chemo-resistant cancer cells outweighed the risk of giving them an agent that could not meet a traditional phase two benchmark. "At a certain point you have to be willing to make a leap," says Dr. Kleinerman. "You have to be willing to take that step off the diving board."

But in 1989, no one in POG wanted to go out onto the diving board again; they had been out on it a few years earlier with MIOS, the Multi-Institutional Osteosarcoma Study. Once was enough.

After the POG meeting, MTP might well have passed into oblivion but for Dr. Paul Meyers of Memorial Sloan-Kettering Cancer Center. Dr. Meyers had served as an adviser to Dr. Kleinerman on the MTP phase two study. And like her, he felt that chemotherapy had taken OS as far up cure mountain as it could. "The fact that all the current OS regimens were achieving approximately the same survival rate indicated a natural ceiling for chemo," he says. "I felt if we were going to save the 35 to 40 percent of kids we were still losing, we had to go in a new direction, take a new avenue."

In 1991, Dr. Meyers's organization, the Children's Cancer Group (CCG), agreed to test MTP, but not alone; it would be incorporated into a major phase three trial already in the planning stage. The centerpiece of this trial was Ifosfamide, a traditional chemotherapy agent.

The CCG board decided that Dr. Meyers, already principal investigator for the Ifosfamide trial, would run the combined Ifosfamide-MTP phase three study. Dr. Kleinerman was sent back to Houston and her lab bench. About the CCG board's decision, she is philosophical. "I don't necessarily care that everyone knows it was my idea. My interest has always been getting this drug out into the real world, and I am extremely grateful to Dr. Meyers for giving me an opportunity to do that."

Dr. Meyers, a veteran of four other phase three trials, says now that 0133 "was the hardest, the most controversial research project I have ever been associated with. There were many times when I was sure the study was going to go down the tubes."

The principal objection of Meyers's critics was and remains that MTP, a drug with no demonstrable tumor-killing power, is being given to untreated patients. Drs. Meyers, Kleinerman, and Fidler might believe that MTP requires a different, perhaps more lenient standard, but is it fair—is it ethical?—to ask a parent to bet her child's best hope, maybe her child's *only* hope, of cure on a drug that cannot shrink a cancer mass?

"Everyone in 0133 is getting a good treatment," counters Dr. Meyers. He notes that even the standard therapy, the therapy Romy received: surgery plus a pre- and postoperative course of three-drug chemo—has a cure rate between 60 and 65 percent. Everyone else is getting the standard therapy *plus* MTP and/or Ifosfamide.

Just before 0133's start, one final change was made. The NCI "invited" POG member institutions to contribute 200 patients to the study. CCG study 7921 became Intergroup study 0133.

As of now only the 0133 Data Monitoring Committee—the group of experts who receive data from all participating hospitals and medical centers—knows what is happening to the kids in each of the study's four arms.

The results of 0133 will not be publicly released until sometime around the turn of the century.

CHAPTER SIX

"WE'RE BAAAAACK."

Two young women in top hats, tails, and oversized shoes were standing in the doorway. The shorter woman, the one with the red nose and curly black hair, looked like Harpo Marx.

"Hello, hello, hello to you," she sang. Her partner joined in. Romy put down her book and smiled . . . slowly. She did not want to be encouraging; otherwise the clowns, two actresses from a downtown theater troupe, might invite themselves into her room. Popular with the little kids on the floor, the clowns annoyed Romy. At fourteen, she felt beyond the charms of baggy pants and funny hats. Besides, their relentless cheerfulness was unsettling. They were like some awful friend who smiles all the time, even when something terrible happens. Their happy talk succeeded only in reminding Romy of how bad she felt, and now, in the middle of November, she did not need any added reminders of that.

The first chemo had made the pain in her knee go away, but that was about the only good thing it did. Romy had been nauseated and feverish since the beginning of October. The worst, though, were the large, red, cankerlike sores inside her mouth and throat.

The short clown asked Romy how she was feeling today.

"A little tired," Romy said; gingerly, she sat up. Four separate leads, from four separate IV bags, were plugged into her chest Broviac this morning. She did not want to disturb them.

The clown knew not to press. "Okay, young lady, you get to rest this time. But we'll be baaack." Romy felt a pang of guilt—she hoped she had not been rude—then closed her eyes. Sleep was the only place that offered her any peace now.

In early November, other signs of depression had also appeared. Romy refused to leave her room, to socialize with the other kids on the floor, to eat. Robin Goodman, the staff psychologist, wanted to call in a psychiatrist. Dr. Rausen was, if not more sanguine, then perhaps more realistic about Romy's mental state. When Pam mentioned Robin Goodman's recommendation, he shrugged and said, "Romy has reason to be depressed. She'll come around. The mind needs time to heal, too."

Romy's own opinion about her mental health was that it was beside the point. Vomiting four or five times a day, coping with constant mouth and throat pain and near-chronic fever absorbed all her energy; she had none to spare for anything else, including other kids. She was even too physically ill to be upset about the change in her appearance.

Always thin, Romy was now almost skeletal. Her weight, 108 in September, had dropped to 94 pounds; and her hair, her wonderful long blond hair, was just about gone now. Romy's long jaw, always prominent, was the first thing you noticed when you met her—that and her skin, which, having lost all its youthful luster, was now cement gray. This combination of changes—the gray, sallow complexion; the thin wisps of hair; the long, serious face—gave Romy the air of a Talmudic scholar.

In mid-October, Romy's aunt, Amy Hochman, gave Romy a

Tweety Bird doll. The doll became a kind of talisman. It went wherever Romy went: into the doughnut hole of the C/T machine, into the ICU. But Tweety was Romy's sole concession to her status as a cancer patient: she avoided the backward-turned baseball cap, the locket of lost hair, all the other paraphernalia the folks on the six o'clock news love to talk about when they do specials on "cancer kids." This attitude alarmed some of the adults around Romy; "this proves she's deeply depressed," they said. But Romy said no, the "cancer kid" mementos just seemed stupid and sentimental to her; maybe they helped other kids, but they did not help her.

Romy's opaque personality makes it hard to know what she was really thinking in late 1994, but one day, when an acquaintance asked her how she felt about her disease, she mentioned a conversation she had had recently with her father.

"A couple of days ago, my dad said to me, 'Boy, Rom, the last few months have been really rough for you.' " Romy paused and looked at the acquaintance. "I told him, 'The last few months, Dad?' I mean when everything happens to you, it makes you think."

One night, about a week after this exchange, Romy awoke with a terrible burning sensation in her chest. She sat up and took a deep breath. *"Owwww!"* It felt as if someone had plunged a red-hot knife into her lungs. She put her hands on her chest and held them there until the pain subsided; then she tried to breathe again. This time, she took a very shallow breath. That helped. Baby breaths eased the pain.

Pam was curled up in a chair at the foot of the bed.

"Mom . . . Mom . . ."

Someone was whispering. Pam opened one eye, then the other. Romy was sitting up in the bed.

"Rom." Pam swung her legs off the arm of the chair; she was facing Romy now. "Are you okay, hon?"

"My lungs are burning. Owww!" Talking hurt. Too much oxygen. Romy's voice dropped to a hoarse whisper. "Can you call a nurse?"

In a minute, a nurse was probing Romy's back with a stethoscope.

"Aaahh, that hurts." Romy jackknifed forward in the bed.

"Sorry, honey." The nurse removed the stethoscope from Romy's back and told her to roll down her smock.

"She has an arrhythmia," Pam said. "She's subject to PVCs [premature ventricular contractions]."

The resident who appeared next asked Romy to roll up her smock again. He took a stethoscope out of his jacket pocket and looked at Pam. "She's subject to PVCs?"

"Yes. I already told the nurse that. Can't you do something? She's in pain."

Romy was still sitting up in bed with the smock pulled up over her head. Pam could hear her breathing in short little gasps.

Another resident came into the room. "A cardiac emergency?"

"Please, can someone call Dr. Rausen?" Pam was surprised at how loud she sounded.

Dr. Rausen, reached at home, identified the source of Romy's pain immediately. She was having a one-in-fifty-thousand reaction to one of her chemotherapeutic agents, methotrexate. Occasionally, very, very occasionally, the drug burns the epithelial cells along the wall of the lungs. In terms of physiological discomfort, the effect is akin to putting a lit match against naked skin, except the lit match is inside the lungs.

The resident who spoke to Dr. Rausen came back into the room, took a syringe out of his pocket, and plunged it into a vial of morphine.

As the cylinder below the needle filled with clear fluid, Romy began to whimper, "No, no, no."

"What's the matter?" the resident asked.

"She's afraid of needles," Pam said. "Rom, it'll only hurt for a minute."

Even in extremis, Romy remained adamant. She shook her head and said no again.

One of the nurses suggested oral morphine. "She'll take a pill, won't she?"

"She can't swallow," Pam said. "She has mouth sores."

Finally, at 5 A.M., three hours after the crisis began, Pam told one of the residents to crush up a half-dozen Percodan pills into powder. "We can spoon-feed the powder to her. She should be able to swallow that."

And fifteen minutes later, sleep came and rescued Romy.

The man was big and lumbering, with pale blue eyes, the palest blue eyes Pam had ever seen. He stood up and wrapped his hands around the back of the chair in front of him. Pam wondered whether the man was nervous, or afraid he would fall if he tried to stand unsupported.

"I'm Michael X. Moriarty," the man said.

Including Pam, there were about two dozen people crowded into a small staff library on the ninth floor, the site of tonight's parents' support group meeting. Moriarty paused. Pam noticed that he was swaying back and forth now. "I think most of you knew Jimmy."

About a dozen people nodded.

"Yesterday was the first anniversary of his death."

No one said anything.

"I've come tonight," Moriarty announced, "to tell you what Kate and I learned over the past two years. Maybe it can help some of you." But Michael Moriarty was really here to console Moriarty, the inconsolable. For the next quarter of an hour, he talked about what a good son James Moriarty had been. How thoughtful and smart and talented Jimmy was, how many things Jimmy could have been if only he had been allowed to live long enough to be them.

Everyone in the room who had known Jimmy Moriarty knew what a good and wonderful boy he had been; lovely Jimmy with his fine, handsome Irish face and soft, sly laugh and sweetness; a sweetness so wonderful it had seemed like God's grace made palpable.

"I had a lot of dreams for Jimmy," Michael said. "He was going to play in the NFL, he was going to be a lawyer, he was going to be president. But when he died, I realized how screwed up my thinking was.

Jimmy wasn't put on earth to fulfill my dreams. No kid is here to fulfill a parent's dreams. We're here to fulfill our kids' dreams."

The next speaker, a woman, said she did not know if anyone else had a similar experience, but sometimes she found herself crying for no reason.

"I just burst into tears. I feel like it's my fault. What's happened to Sarah."

"Guilt is a very common emotion for parents," said the young social worker leading the meeting. "It's normal to feel what you're feeling, Mrs. Lowenthal."

The consolation sounded tinny to Pam, but, she thought, what else could the social worker say? What could anyone say to the people in this room?

The woman was still talking. Like Michael Moriarty, she had gotten lost in her own grief. "I could always fix Sarah's boo-boos. When she was little, I'd put a Band-Aid on them, give them a kiss. And they'd go away. Sarah thought she had a magic mommy. That's what she use to call me, Magic Mommy. She thought I could make anything go away."

People began to turn their heads. It seemed indecent to look upon this kind of suffering.

When the woman sat down, the social worker introduced the featured speaker, an OS survivor, a thirty-two-year-old woman who had gotten the disease in 1980 and survived a 1982 relapse, which was roughly the equivalent of surviving two plane crashes. A pair of crutches were leaning on the table between the social worker and the speaker. Pam looked under the table; the young woman's right leg was missing.

"I don't think I can listen to any more of this," Pam said to Debbie Norberg, the woman she had come to the meeting with.

Debbie was the mother who had been hovering over the swollen pink ball on the gurney in the pediatric ICU in October. A few days after the encounter, a nurse told Pam that Debbie's little boy Peter was under observation in the east wing. "They think he's got leukemia," the nurse said, as she checked Romy's IV tubing, "but no one knows what kind. They're doing tests now." Two weeks later, Debbie told Pam the rest of Peter's story herself.

In the middle of September, he had come home from nursery school with a sore throat; the family doctor said it was a cold. But the next day, a fever developed; a few days later, listlessness. Suddenly, five-year-old Peter was too tired to watch television, too tired to walk to the bathroom, too tired to do anything but sleep. Small waves of fear began to wash over Debbie. Peter had had colds before, but never like this.

At the end of September, Peter woke up with a small, perfectly shaped golf ball behind each ear. Grotesquely swollen, his glands were now almost perfect spheres. "Your son's in kidney failure," an ER doctor told Debbie. But no one at the Staten Island hospital knew why Peter had gone into kidney failure or how to reverse it. It was as if the little boy had become the victim of an awful cosmic prank, as if someone had hooked up his little body to an invisible helium machine. All through the day and into the night, Peter's arms, face, and legs expanded, grew bigger and bigger, became more and more swollen, more and more bloated.

The next morning, the noisy *whack whack* of a landing helicopter woke Debbie in the hospital lounge. She was sipping a cup of cold coffee when a doctor came in and told her to put on her coat. An ambulance helicopter was on the roof. The helicopter would take her and Peter across New York Harbor to NYU Medical Center.

Leukemia was still the working diagnosis when Pam and Debbie met in late October, but the doctors were having trouble identifying which of the several different types of pediatric leukemia Peter had.

"Acute lymphocyte leukemia is everybody's current favorite, now," Debbie said on the elevator down from the support group meeting. In the lobby, the women buttoned their coats and walked out to the courtyard.

Pam and Debbie, the only two smokers on the floor, had met in the courtyard three weeks earlier on a cigarette break. The mutual breaks, serendipitous at first, quickly developed into mutual support sessions.

Pam admired funny, energetic, soulful Debbie; she also envied Debbie's exuberant in-your-face style.

One morning, walking to the elevators, Pam found her dressing down a pretty young nurse about the pediatric ICU rest room.

"It's unbelievably unsanitary in there," Debbie was complaining. "It's a pigsty. You should be ashamed of yourself. The hospital should be ashamed of itself." Debbie stopped when she saw Pam. "Aren't I right, Pam? Isn't the bathroom in there a mess? Jesus, you could get the clap in there! Tell Snow White here."

Debbie was right about the hideous state of the ICU bathroom. It was an eyesore. But the nurses were the empresses of the ninth floor. Offend one and you might not get your calls answered as promptly. Pam decided to be diplomatic.

"Honestly, it could use a cleaning."

The young woman nodded and promised to talk to the maintenance staff.

A few days later, the nurse stopped Pam in the hall. "Well, Miss Staten Island's been a busy girl, hasn't she?"

Pam asked who Miss Staten Island was.

"Your friend Debbie," the nurse said. "This morning she took it upon herself to clean the ICU bathroom." After the nurse left, Pam slipped into the bathroom. It was now miraculously clean. On the outside door, a sign warned: PARENTS, THIS IS OUR BATHROOM, PLEASE KEEP IT CLEAN. Another sign over the sink admonished visitors: PLEASE PICK UP AFTER YOURSELF.

"Well, if it isn't Mrs. Clean herself," Pam said the next morning in the courtyard.

"*Ms.* Clean, honey," Debbie replied and began to giggle. "That'll teach Snow White, won't it? The uptight little shit."

More than anything else, though, what drew Pam to Debbie was Debbie's sheer, unreasoning certainty; her absolute conviction that Peter would be all right. Pam knew that the certainty was a form of craziness. No one in Debbie's position (or Pam's) could be certain of anything. But it did not matter. On the ninth floor, you took hope wherever you could find it.

Even when pediatric leukemia was eliminated as a possible diagnosis, Debbie remained unreasoningly hopeful.

"Now the docs are completely clueless," she told Pam in the courtyard one night in early December. The two women were huddled in a corner near the lobby; it was the only place that offered any protection from the biting wind. Through the plate-glass window, Pam could see workmen putting up Christmas decorations in the reception area.

"How are you doing?" she asked Debbie.

"Me? Scared shitless. But I believe that as long as I believe Peter's going to be all right, Peter *will* be all right. It's part of my deal with God. Don't you feel the same way about Romy?"

The thought had not occurred to Pam before, but she looked at Debbie and said, "Yes. I do."

CHAPTER SEVEN

CLINICAL TRIALS VARY CONSIDERABLY IN CHARACTER. IN AIDS THEY often resemble jazz pieces: wild, improvisational, hot, full of inspired solos. Cancer trials, especially big phase three trials, are more like major symphony pieces. Each movement of the study unfolds at a stately, orderly, magisterial pace.

A few weeks before Christmas, Romy was prepared for the second movement of 0133: surgical removal of her tumor. One day in the middle of the month, she was slid inside a C/T machine in the radiology department and her much-photographed knee was photographed some more. The results would show how much, if any at all, the first round of chemotherapy had shrunk the tumor on the knee.

One morning a few days later, Pam heard the quick pitter-patter of footsteps outside Romy's room. The sound was as rhythmic as a dance step. When she looked up, Dr. Rausen was standing in the doorway.

"Hi, Dr. Rausen."

"Good morning to you, Mrs. Hochman." The physician bowed slightly.

Dr. Rausen carried around so many facts in his head, sometimes he forgot what he had come to tell you. This morning was one of those times. Pam had to remind him of the scan results.

"Ah, yes, Romy's scan results. The results were inconclusive, Mrs. Hochman. The tumor is as big now as it was in October."

Dr. Rausen quickly added that this was not as alarming as it sounded. "Scan results don't necessarily mean anything good or bad, Mrs. Hochman. We had hoped to see shrinkage, but a dying tumor doesn't always shrink, sometimes the dead cells stick together. When the surgeon inspects the tumor visually next month, we'll have a clearer picture. One good sign, though . . ." Dr. Rausen looked at Romy, who was eyeing him intently from the bed. "The pain. It's a good sign that the pain is gone."

"She doesn't eat, she isn't leaving her room. . . ." It was twenty minutes later, and Pam was standing in the hall telling Dr. Rausen about Romy's continuing emotional deterioration.

"I know, I know. I can see how bad she is," he said. Then he told Pam that Romy was probably going to lose her leg.

Pam's hands suddenly began to flutter wildly. For a moment, she thought she was going to lift off, fly right through the ceiling. "Did you see a new complication in the scan?"

Dr. Rausen shook his head. The problem was positioning. Sometimes a tumor becomes so enmeshed in the surrounding blood vessels that extraction is impossible, so the leg has to be removed, too. "We couldn't tell much about the artery-vein placement from the scan," he said. "But there's a possibility that could happen with Romy."

Pam was angry now. In September, Dr. Rausen had promised that Romy would keep her leg. Well, no, as she thought about it, he had not been quite that definite; he had said Romy would probably keep her leg. "I wasn't expecting this," Pam said. "I wasn't expecting this at all." She had folded her hands across her chest to stop the fluttering.

Dr. Rausen bowed slightly. "I'm sorry, Mrs. Hochman, I didn't mean to upset you. I have another patient. I hope you'll understand."

That night Pam spent a lot of time thinking about Aaron Rausen. Underneath the formal exterior and ever-present gray suit, he was a good and decent man, but his decency had an element of obtuseness to it. Maybe not obtuseness, Pam thought, maybe self-protectiveness. She did not blame Dr. Rausen for that. In his line of work, you had to be protective; otherwise you would get your heart broken every day. Still, he could be a little more sensitive, a little more careful about delivering bad news.

Just before Christmas, the Hochmans had a visit from Donald Pearlman, the surgeon who had biopsied Romy's knee in September and who would perform the surgery in January.

Dr. Pearlman was even more pessimistic about the leg than Dr. Rausen. The surgeon said a definitive diagnosis would have to await a visual inspection of the tumor. But as of now, Romy's odds of keeping the leg were only fifty-fifty. "If the tumor is near a big artery, I'll have to take the leg, too."

"You'll do it right then?" Pam asked. "The amputation."

"Right then, or if you prefer, we can wait a week. Some kids adjust better if they have a little time to prepare themselves for the loss."

A week to say good-bye to your leg: This struck Pam as an awful option.

Dr. Pearlman had one other piece of news. The surgery would be done at his hospital, the Hospital for Joint Diseases, on January 13. After he left, Jack checked his datebook. "Oh shit," he said. "You know what day the thirteenth is? It's a Friday. Romy's going to have the operation on Friday the thirteenth."

"Fifty-fifty," Romy said the next day. "That's what Pearlman said? I thought Rausen said I could keep my leg. I remember him saying that in the conference room in September. I don't understand."

Pam put her hand on top of Romy's. "Rausen said 'probably,' Rom."

"You know what I think?" Jack said. He was standing at the foot of the bed. "I think Pearlman does this on purpose. He tells you the absolute worst that can happen, so he'll look like a big hero when the worst doesn't happen. Our friend Dr. Pearlman is no dummy."

"Do you think I'll be able to keep my leg, Mom?"

Pam wanted to shout, "Yes, of course! What a silly question!" But the best she could do was: "We'll just have to wait and see, hon."

Later, out in the hall, Jack got mad when Pam said it would be terrible if Pearlman had to amputate. "Jesus," he yelled at her, "don't talk like that! Don't even *think* like that. Romy's not going to lose her leg, you hear me? She's not." Then he spun around and stomped off.

The morning of Friday, January 13, was brilliantly sunny and very cold. Pam finished buttoning her coat, a heavy tan shepherd's jacket, then picked up the remote from the bed and pressed the off button. The TV screen went dark.

Outside in the hall two boys were standing next to the elevators, discussing cancer medications.

The older boy said he was starting a new regimen next week. Phenylalanine mustard plus cyclophosphamide.

The younger one nodded and said that phenylalanine mustard was like one of the drugs he was taking: actinomycin D.

The boys pronounced the names of the drugs perfectly.

Pam looked at them. In September, she would have found this conversation surreal. Now, after two months at Ronald McDonald, she was used to everything, even baby oncologists.

There were still men working at the construction site across from the Hospital for Joint Diseases. A dozen workers in bright yellow-and-blue hats were gathered around an oil drum with a fire in it when Pam got out of the cab. On this bitterly cold morning, the men had the grim end-of-the-line look of a gulag work party. Pam checked her watch:

eleven o'clock, still a little time. She walked down to Seventeenth Street and bought a hot dog from a vendor. As she ate, she looked back at the site. White smoke from a steam pump was billowing up over the yellow-and-blue hats into a clear, sharp winter sky.

Upstairs, the Levines and the Hochmans had assembled in a twelfth-floor waiting room like two wary armies. Pam's father and mother, Ben and Annette Levine, were seated by a window; the Hochmans—George, Jack's father, and Amy and Jack—were around a portable metal table near the exit on the opposite side. The room was full of ancient ironies, but Pam was too preoccupied to be troubled by them this morning. She smiled at Amy. Amy smiled back, but George Hochman avoided her glance. George blamed Pam for everything: for the drugs, for Jack's bankruptcy, probably even for Romy's cancer.

"Mr. and Mrs. Hochman."

Dr. Pearlman was standing in the doorway. The loose gray-green surgical suit made his squat frame look even squatter.

"Can I have a word with you, please?"

Pam walked over to the doorway: "We get to see Romy before she goes in, don't we?"

Dr. Pearlman ignored the question. "If I know right away that I'm going to have to amputate, the surgery will be relatively short, about three hours. If I can save the leg, it'll be longer; somewhere between six to six and a half hours. Her chances of keeping the leg are fifty-fifty."

"Can we see Romy?" Pam asked again.

Dr. Pearlman smiled. "Sure. She's down on the tenth floor."

On the elevator, Pam could feel the hot dog coming back on her. For a moment, she thought she was going to vomit; the nausea passed.

Romy, glassy-eyed and pale, was lying on a gurney outside the operating room. Pam bent down and kissed her. "She's been sedated," Dr. Pearlman said. He was standing at the head of the gurney. Jack slipped his hand under Romy's and bent down. "How's my little girl?" he whispered. "Everything is going to be all right, you'll see. All right?"

Pam felt another spike of nausea. She took a deep breath.

A masked figure emerged from the operating room. "Doctor, it's noon. We're ready now."

Just before vanishing inside, Dr. Pearlman reminded the Hochmans a final time of Romy's odds.

"Maybe he ought to change his name to Dr. Fifty-fifty," Jack said.

Pam started to smile, then stopped. "I'm going to vomit," she said and ran to the ladies' room.

The next several hours had a gauzy, slightly unreal feel to them. Pam vomited twice more; then, around two, she began to seesaw back and forth between chills and profuse sweating. An hour later, her shoulders began to shake; Jack got a blanket and wrapped it around her, then he went out to the nurses' station to see if Pearlman had called.

"Nothing," he said when he came back.

At four, there was still no word.

Finally, at four-thirty, a nurse appeared in the waiting room. Dr. Pearlman wanted the Hochmans on the tenth floor right away.

"Four and half hours," Jack said on the way to the elevator. "That's midway between three and six. What do you think it means?"

Pam said she didn't know.

On ten, everything happened very quickly. An excited Dr. Pearlman met them at the elevator. "Yes, yes," he said, "Romy's fine; we were able to save the leg." He grabbed Pam's hand and led her into a small changing room. "The tumor was entirely necrotized, Mrs. Hochman; here, you both have to put on a surgical gown."

"It was dead?" Pam asked; she took the surgical gown from Dr. Pearlman.

"Uh-huh, I could peel the tumor off the bone. I didn't have to cut at all. We were able to insert a prosthesis easily. Here . . ." The surgeon handed Pam a funny green hat like the one he was wearing. "That's a very unusual result, Mrs. Hochman, a very good sign. Here, you have to wear this, too." Dr. Pearlman wrapped the surgical mask around her face. "We didn't even need to create a skin flap to protect the surgical wound against infection."

"That's good? That's unusual, too?"

"Very unusual." The surgeon took Pam's hand again and led her through a set of doors. Jack was right behind them.

In the recovery room, the surgeon stopped in front of a bed surrounded by IV poles. Romy lay semiconscious under the canopy of steel and plastic.

"She's the color of stone!" Pam exclaimed.

"She's lost a lot of blood," Dr. Pearlman said. "We're transfusing her now."

Pam walked over to the bed and bent down. "Rom . . . hon, you know you're okay. You have your leg. Can you understand me? You have your leg."

Romy seemed too weak and drugged to understand anything; but when a nurse walked over to check the IV tubing, her eyes suddenly opened and she shouted, "No needles, *no needles, please.*"

Pam began to laugh, then to cry.

Dr. Pearlman smiled. "Your daughter certainly has an aversion to needles. She's said the same thing to every nurse who's gotten near her."

Ben and Annette Levine were standing on the other side of the glass partition next to Romy's bed. Pam smiled and gave them the thumbs-up sign.

Just then, Romy bolted upright in the bed and vomited.

Maybe it was a sympathetic reaction, but Pam felt a surge of nausea.

"I think I'm going to be sick again," she said.

Jack smiled at her. "You look worse than Romy. Why don't you go back to Ronald McDonald? Amy will stay with us."

"You're sure?"

"I'm sure."

On the way out of the recovery room, Pam ran into the surgeon who had assisted Dr. Pearlman. "It went wonderfully well," he said. "Now she'll be able to get on with her life. You all will."

The next morning Pam woke up very sick, but very happy. The leg was saved, the tumor, dead and gone; and the Hochmans, she and Jack, had been a very good, very effective team yesterday. From here on out, it was all downhill. Physical therapy for the knee; a second round of post-operative chemotherapy; then in August, after the chemo, L.A. and the start of a new life together. Romy and Pam. Mother and daughter.

A week after Romy's surgery, Peter Norberg's illness was finally diagnosed.

Peter had Burkitt's lymphoma, a very rare form of lymph cancer. "It's sort of like getting into Harvard," Debbie said one brilliantly sunny morning in the courtyard. "Except that it's even harder than getting into Harvard; only about three hundred kids a year get it. How many kids do you think there are in America, Pam? Fifty million? And three hundred get it. Three hundred and Peter." Debbie stopped and took a drag of her cigarette. "Only three percent of kids survive."

Pam put her hand on Debbie's arm.

"He's not going to die, Pam. Peter's not going to die."

"I know he isn't." Pam put her other arm around Debbie and hugged her.

CHAPTER EIGHT

In October, Paul Gertz had told Pam that his son Daniel and Daniel's friend Justin Gitlin, another 0133 subject, had spent only five days a month at the medical center; three days at the beginning of each chemotherapy cycle and two days at the end of it. "That's about typical for study kids," Paul had said. But chemo made Romy so sick she left NYU only twice during her first five months in trial 0133. In November, she had Thanksgiving dinner at Pam's Ronald McDonald House apartment on East Seventy-third Street, and in January, after the surgery, she spent a celebratory weekend there.

She and Pam rented *Sleepless in Seattle* and *Thelma and Louise* and gorged themselves on take-out Chinese and pizza (for the first time in months, Romy actually had an appetite); they gossiped, they told each other bad jokes, they dished the doctors and nurses, and they talked about the future. About how different life would be once life began again in California in eight months. The last evening of the weekend, Romy took out a map of Los Angeles, opened it, and searched the reference points until she found the spot where Wilshire Boulevard begins near the beach in Santa Monica.

Romy put her finger on the spot and pushed it eastward across the face of the map through Westwood, Beverly Hills, and Fairfax; at Hancock Park, her finger stopped. Hancock Park was where she and Pam would live in L.A. What did she know about Hancock Park? Romy knew that Nat King Cole used to live there; Pam had told her that a few weeks earlier, but Romy did not know who Nat King Cole was.

Next, Romy looked for Arden Boulevard. That was the name of the street she and Pam were going to live on; they were going to share a house on Arden with her aunt Lisa and her uncle James and their new baby, Anna. According to the map, the street was a few blocks north of Wilshire. Romy put her finger on the street marked Arden, and closed her eyes. What did Arden Boulevard look like? The first thing Romy saw were palm trees, enormously tall palm trees, dozens of them running at intervals along a broad, stately avenue. Next, she saw homes, large Spanish-style homes with tiled roofs; each bordered by bougainvillea and set on a broad swath of lovely green lawn that rose gently up from the sidewalk. This was what Lisa's house looked like in photographs; it was an absolutely sensational house, Romy thought. Large but not imposing, handsome but homey—the perfect house for a big happy California family.

Next, she tried to imagine what the Hancock Park High kids would be like. Probably great-looking; California kids always were great-looking, tanned, with terrific bodies. This worried Romy. She finally felt well enough to be concerned about her appearance. She was very bald and very pale and very thin, and since chemo did not end until August, she would probably be very bald and very pale and very thin when school started in September. On the other hand, she would be walking by then. According to Dr. Pearlman, she might be walking even sooner.

Romy took a pencil and notepad from the nightstand and made a list of things she would need to do before the start of school. Buy a new wardrobe—that was the most important thing. None of her old clothes fit anymore, and besides, they were Smithtown clothes. She would need a different kind of wardrobe for Hancock Park. California clothes. She also would have to buy makeup. Her mother could help her with that. Pam knew everything there was to know about clothes and makeup.

Owww. Romy felt a stinging sensation in her knee. She put the pencil down and began to massage the knee, gently. Her memory of the surgery was very hazy. She recalled Dr. Pearlman saying, "This looks very good," and she remembered shouting, "No needles, please!" and vomiting a lot. But everything else was a blank. She did not remember seeing Pam and Jack in the recovery room or asking the nurses if she still had her leg. Romy rubbed the knee again very carefully.

The rest of her stay at Joint Diseases had been uneventful, except for the day the bandages were changed for the first time. There was a big, ugly blister on top of the surgical wound; Dr. Pearlman seemed surprised by it. He poked and probed at the blister delicately with a gloved finger, then turned to Romy, who was sitting up on the examining table. He told her to brace herself. He was going to have to pull the rest of the bandage off; "It's going to hurt," he said.

Romy, an expert on pain, asked how much it was going to hurt.

Dr. Pearlman promised to rip off the bandage quickly.

Romy nodded, shut her eyes tightly, and gripped the sides of the table.

"Ready?" Dr. Pearlman asked.

"Ready," someone else said.

A ripping sound, then searing pain. Romy screamed. When she opened her eyes again, a sticky greenish fluid was oozing from a hole in her knee. The next day a resident told Pam a skin flap should have been placed over the incision, as originally planned. The blister had formed because the skin around the wound was too tight; a flap would have facilitated healing by easing some of the pressure.

There was a jingling noise outside the door. Romy looked up from her knee toward the door. Someone was fumbling through a purse. Pam must be looking for her keys. "It's open, Mom." Romy picked up the map from the bed and folded it neatly. Pam walked in with their dinner.

"I got your favorite." Pam reached into the bag and removed a white container.

"Spicy Amazing Chicken?" Romy asked.

"Not only that . . ." Pam removed another white container from the bag and held it up.

"General Liu's Mad Pork." She made a little bow. General Liu's Mad Pork was a special favorite of Romy's.

After dinner, mother and daughter watched television until eleven, when the last of their favorite shows, *ER,* ended. Then they talked until around one, when Pam, still woozy from the flu, fell asleep.

A single tumor slice, a slice thinner even than a candy wafer, is used to assess a tumor's overall state of decay and degeneration. If 70 percent of the cells in the slice are dead, the patient receives a 70 percent cell kill because it is assumed that 70 percent of the cells in the tumor are also dead. The day after Romy's tumor was removed, it was sent to a medical center laboratory, where a pathologist cut off a small slice of the now calcified growth and slid it under a microscope. The next afternoon, the pathologist called Dr. Rausen's office. Twenty minutes later, Dr. Rausen asked his secretary, Janice Pelt, to call the Hochmans at the medical center.

Pam was curled up in a chair next to Romy's bed when the phone rang.

"Hello, Romy Hochman's room."

"Mrs. Hochman, is that you?" The voice on the other end, liquid and gravelly, sounded surprised.

"Hi, Dr. Rausen."

"Mrs. Hochman . . ." There was still a question mark in the voice.

"It's me, Dr. Rausen. Honest."

"I've never heard your voice on the phone before, Mrs. Hochman. Do you realize that? We've never talked on the phone."

Pam smiled. Sometimes, Dr. Rausen's directness was almost child-like. Suddenly another less happy thought intruded. Rausen had seen Romy this morning. Why would he be calling the room now, at supper time? Pam asked him if anything was wrong.

"Wrong? No, nothing is wrong." Pam could almost see Dr. Rausen shaking his head. "Just the opposite, in fact, Mrs. Hochman. Good news. Very good news." The physician said he had just received Romy's cell kill analysis. She had 100 percent cell kill. In oncology, Dr. Rausen declared, 100 percent was as close as anyone ever got to a complete cure. Ninety-five percent of patients with 100 percent kills were still alive ten years later. One hundred was a very uncommon score. Only about 20 percent of the children in trial 0133 got it.

"Is Romy there?" he asked. "I'd like to tell her the good news myself."

Pam said that Romy was taking a nap.

"Oh." Dr. Rausen sounded disappointed. "Well, I'll be in in the morning to talk to her."

"So we're out of the woods now?" Pam noticed that she was speaking very loudly.

"Romy is as cured as she can be," Dr. Rausen said.

What did that mean, Pam wondered as she hung up. That Romy was cured or as cured as anyone with OS could be? The language of oncology had a Houdini-like slipperiness to it; even the most irrevocable, the most straightforward of statements often contained secret escape routes.

"Cured as she can be," Pam decided, means cured if you had an honest tumor.

One of the most amazing things about the ninth floor was the sensitivity of its grapevine. People seemed to know about a thing the moment it occurred. Pam could never figure out how this happened. Sometimes, she half thought, all the pain, all the suffering on the floor created a kind of ether, a heavier-than-air atmosphere that transmitted news instantly from person to person, room to room. The night Dr. Rausen phoned, the grapevine was operating especially well.

The moment Romy woke up, Kelly Cervone and Gail Garrity, two of her favorite nurses, appeared in the room to offer congratulatory hugs; next, the nutritionist stopped by. Another big hug. Then a few of the parents drifted in. More hugs. The biggest hug of all came from Paul Gertz. Paul said a nurse in the radiology department told him about Romy's cell kill. He was waiting for Daniel; Daniel was having his first posttrial monitoring scan this afternoon.

"One hundred percent, that's wonderful," Paul said. "I'm very happy for you, really." He smiled. "And you know what? You beat us. Daniel only got a 93 percent kill."

The "beat us" bothered Pam. Sometimes, good news had a strange effect on other parents. They smiled, they congratulated you, they told you how happy they were for you, but often when they walked away, they were thinking, Why couldn't it have been my child? Why couldn't *he* be the one with the perfect score?

Not that Pam blamed them. Last fall, watching Daniel and the other kids in trial 0133 breeze in and out of the medical center, she had felt just as jealous, just as resentful. Still, Paul's reaction made her uneasy.

That night, Pam promised herself that unless someone asked, she would keep Romy's score to herself.

The next morning, Dr. Rausen stopped by the room to offer his congratulations. He told Romy how uncommon her cell kill was and how happy he was for her. Then he delivered one of his elliptical non sequiturs. "Unlike some other people," he said, "you won't be coming back here." Later, one of the nurses deciphered this Rausenism for the Hochmans. The previous day, the nurse said, Daniel Gertz's friend Justin Gitlin had been admitted to the medical center with a relapse.

This was the first bad news Romy heard about a fellow trial member, but it was not the last.

Lotte Kauffman, Romy's first roommate, had been in 0133; she was in Arm B: Ifosfamide, plus cisplatin, Adriamycin, and methotrexate, the same arm as Daniel Gertz. But Lotte had gotten no succor from the drugs; her OS, indomitable and insatiable, took her leg, and then immediately went after her lungs. In October, when Romy met her, Lotte was in the hospital to have several small cancerous pulmonary growths removed. A brief period of peace and well-being followed the surgery. Over the fall and very early winter, the Lotte news that floated through the ninth-floor ether was generally good. Lotte was finally in remission, Lotte was applying to college, Lotte was planning a trip to Israel this summer, Lotte had gained seven pounds, Lotte was beginning to look like her old self. Then suddenly, in mid-January, about the time Romy's cell kill count was announced, the Lotte news turned bad again. Lotte was having terrible back pain. Lotte had developed a hacking cough again; Lotte was dying.

In early February, Lotte returned to the ninth floor. "She came in last night," a nurse said as she checked the heart monitor next to Romy's bed. That evening, a young resident brought more news. A C/T scan indicated a spinal metastasis; Lotte was having exploratory surgery on Friday. If the new metastasis was very small and very recent, some kind of treatment might be attempted, but as of now no one was very optimistic.

"I'm giving Lotte a tea party tomorrow afternoon," said the resident, a young woman named Jeanne Lapidus. "I'd like the two of you to come. It's at three in Lotte's room."

"Can we bring anything?" Pam asked.

"Just yourselves and a happy face," Dr. Lapidus said.

Lotte was sitting in the bed wearing lipstick, rouge, a touch of eye shadow, and a bright red bow in her hair when Pam wheeled Romy into the room the next afternoon. Lotte looked sweet and sad, and very sick. Rachel Kauffman, who was sitting next to her daughter on the bed, just looked sad, sad the way Michael Moriarty had looked sad at the parents' support group meeting, sad the way only people on the ninth floor looked sad.

Lotte smiled when she saw Pam and Romy. "Hi, you guys."

Pam wheeled Romy over to the bed; Romy put her hand in Lotte's and squeezed it. Pam leaned down and embraced her.

The small room was crowded; there were about nine other guests. Pam got a piece of cake and went over to the window and squeezed in between a nurse and another parent, a short, blond, pudgy man named David Knox. David and his wife, Christie, were from Akron, Ohio; they were here in New York because of their eight-year-old son, Will. Last year, just before Christmas, healthy, athletic, bubbly, chubby Will began to display a bizarre catalog of symptoms. First, Will had trouble standing up on his Rollerblades, then Will began seeing things double, then Will developed terrible headaches.

In January, doctors in Akron discovered a golf ball–sized tumor on the left side of Will's brain. Three weeks later, the tumor was removed at NYU. Last Saturday, Pam had seen Will for the first time since the surgery; he looked as if he had been whipped across the face with a barbed wire. A scar ran diagonally from the left side of his forehead, down over his eye, to his right ear.

"How are you today, Will?" Pam had asked.

Will had looked right at her, but he didn't say anything; his expression was vacant.

Pam decided she would not ask David about Will this afternoon.

"Picture!" someone shouted. "Picture!" Lotte was sitting up in the bed, Dr. Lapidus was standing at her left, Rachel Kauffman was on her right. All three women were smiling. When the flash of the camera went off, a small child with a bald head, a six- or seven-year-old, clapped her hands and squealed. Other people laughed.

Someone asked Lotte what she was going to major in at college.

"Art history, with a minor in political science."

At about three, the room began to empty out. The mother of the bald child took her daughter across the floor for a chemotherapy session; David Knox left to relieve his wife at Will's bedside; two of the nurses announced that they were due on rounds at three-fifteen. When Pam and Romy left, Lotte was talking to Dr. Lapidus. Rachel Kauffman was sitting on the bed, watching them, watching Lotte.

Saturday evening, there was more Lotte news. A nurse told Romy the surgery did not go well. The doctors found extensive spinal involvement; too extensive for a medical intervention. Lotte's cancer was terminal.

The last piece of Lotte news came on March first, the day before Romy's birthday. Pam was having lunch in the cafeteria on the first floor when Dr. Lapidus, looking very young and very pale, stopped at her table.

Pam knew right away. "Lotte," she said.

"Yesterday afternoon," the resident said.

Just then, an old man in a brightly colored jogging suit walked by the table. At this time of day, the cafeteria looked like a rest stop on an interstate highway in August: jeans, work shirts, warm-up outfits, running shoes, sweatshirts. At the medical center, even the dying dressed for summer vacation.

Pam asked how Lotte's parents were doing.

"All right," Dr. Lapidus said, then amended her statement. "The father's doing all right; the mother isn't."

A few days later, Lotte's hometown newspaper carried a small obituary. It noted that Lotte Kauffman would have been eighteen in July and had planned to attend Brandeis University in the fall.

CHAPTER NINE

In March 1993, Eileen Hochman wrote a farewell letter to her granddaughter Romy. Two days later, Eileen, who had terminal liver cancer, gave the letter to her daughter Amy and asked Amy to present it to Romy on her eighteenth birthday.

In February 1995, Amy decided that Romy should have the letter. "I think we ought to give it to her for her birthday," Amy told Jack one morning. "I'm sure Mom would understand."

Jack liked the idea. Maybe there was something in the letter that Romy needed to hear, something that would lift her spirits, bring her further back into life.

On March second, Romy's fifteenth birthday, Amy drove up to New York to make the presentation.

"I have something for you, Rom," Amy said, after Pam left the room. She sat down on the bed and opened her purse. "It's a letter from Grandmother Eileen. I was supposed to give it to you on your eighteenth birthday. But I think if Mom knew . . ." Amy stopped. She did not want to say the word cancer. "Sometimes Mom talks to me,"

Amy said, "and the other night, she told me that she wanted you to have the letter now. For your birthday." Amy reached into her bag and took out a manila envelope.

Romy took the envelope and put it on the nightstand next to the bed.

"It's a special letter," Amy said. "Grandmother Eileen wanted to tell you how much she loved you."

"I don't want to read it now," Romy said. Then she began to cry.

"It's okay to be sad, Rom. I'm sure Grandmother Eileen would understand. Here . . ." Amy picked up the letter from the nightstand and put it in Romy's lap.

"Get it away from me!" Romy shouted. She pushed the letter off the bed; it landed on the floor next to the Tweety Bird doll. Romy was crying hard.

Amy was angry at herself now. Why had she been so blind? Of course, the letter would upset Romy. She picked it up and put it back in her purse. "I'm sorry, hon. I didn't mean to upset you. We'll save the letter for later. When you're older."

"No," Romy said, shaking her head. "I don't ever want to see it again."

"Never, then. Okay."

Later during a conversation, a friend asked Romy about this incident. Was Amy right? Did Eileen Hochman's letter frighten her?

Romy shrugged and talked around the point. Finally she said, yes, the letter had. "I was sure I'd die if I read it. I can't explain why. But I was sure I would. It was like the letter was a dead person who was reaching out of the grave to pull me in." She began to laugh nervously. "I know it sounds totally weird but that's how I felt."

No, her friend said, it didn't sound weird at all. He would feel the same way. He also reminded Romy that, in a way, her feelings about the letter were right. It had turned out to be an omen, a portent of sorts.

Romy thought about this for a moment, then agreed. Amy's visit . . . the letter . . . did mark a turning point, didn't they?

•   •   •

From the beginning of the year until Amy's visit nothing but good news had flowed into Romy's life; thereafter bad news became the norm again, and the bad news started almost immediately.

On St. Patrick's Day, Romy checked into NYU for the beginning of a new chemotherapy cycle. The next morning, Amy, who was visiting again, came by at nine; when she arrived, Romy said she felt feverish.

Amy walked over to the bed and checked her forehead. It was burning. "I'm going to get a nurse, Rom."

"Morning rounds begin in a few minutes," a nurse at the station told Amy. "Someone will look at her then."

Amy went back into the room and checked Romy's forehead again: hotter now. Could a fever worsen in just two minutes? Amy put her hand on Romy's back. No, it was not her imagination. The skin on Romy's back felt very hot too.

"Good morning." A resident.

Amy was so relieved, she could have kissed him. "Can you take my niece's temperature? I think she has a fever."

The resident shook his head. He did not take temperatures. That was the nurse's job.

Amy asked the resident if he could at least feel Romy's forehead.

He said a nurse would be in in a few minutes, then wrote something down on Romy's chart and left.

"Ooowww, I feel weird." Amy turned around. Romy was sitting up in the bed shivering.

A spike of panic. Amy went over to the doorway and looked into the hall. There was a nurse standing next to a breakfast cart near the elevators. Amy approached her. "Can you help us?" she asked. "My niece is running a very high fever." The nurse told Amy that she was about to go off duty; someone would look in on Romy when morning rounds began. The nurse looked at her watch. Rounds started in ten minutes.

Amy grabbed her by the arm. "Someone needs to look in on my niece *now*."

"Her temperature is 104," the nurse said as she slipped the thermometer back into her pocket. A small knot of worried muscle had formed between the nurse's eyebrows. "I'll be right back," she said, then vanished into the hall. A few seconds later, the ward supervisor appeared. The supervisor took Romy's temperature. It was now 105. At 107, Romy could begin to convulse.

The first nurse reappeared with a second nurse. "Help me undress her," the ward supervisor said.

A white huddle formed around Romy; a smock, panties, and a headband flew into the air. The huddle unscrambled; Romy, naked, dazed, sweaty, and still shivering reappeared on the bed. Amy looked around. The room was full now; there were five or six people—nurses and residents—around the bed. One of the new arrivals, a stocky young man, asked Amy to stand by the wall.

Someone draped a towel over Romy's shoulders; someone else wrapped her legs in a sheet. Another towel went over her head. Now there was a gurney in the room. It was wheeled up to the side of the bed.

"ICU?" one of the nurses asked.

"No," the stocky young resident said. "Radiology. We need to do a C/T scan immediately."

The next day, Romy's condition was diagnosed as *Pneumocystis carinii* pneumonia, a virulent form of pneumonia rarely seen outside AIDS. PCP is associated with a severely compromised immune system, and while chemotherapy can, like HIV, depress the immune system, cases of chemotherapy-related PCP are so rare, Romy's case won her a fleeting moment of medical fame.

A week later, the C/T scan of Romy's lungs was the star attraction at the medical center's grand rounds. A professor challenged the class of residents and interns to identify the cause of the white cloud in the left lung of Patient 106.

"I recognized you right away," a resident told Romy.

Romy asked him how.

Easy, the resident replied. "You were only the second non-AIDS patient to develop PCP at the medical center this year."

At the end of March, news about another 0133 participant reached Romy. Moira Blake. Moira had relapsed in the middle of the month; according to the ninth-floor grapevine, she was returning to the medical center for lung surgery the following week. The next day, Romy and Pam did a little calculation. Of the four 0133 participants on the ninth floor they knew about, one, Lotte, was dead, and two others, Moira and Justin, had relapsed.

Sixty-six percent is a terrible relapse rate, but Romy still had two iron-hard facts to place between herself and her fear: her cell-kill count and Daniel Gertz. If Lotte represented the dark side of OS, what it could do to you, Daniel represented what you could do to OS, how you could stop the disease, defeat it. Romy would say later that, in her mind, Daniel became a talisman. As long as he was all right, she believed she would be all right. And in late March 1995, the news about Daniel continued to be good.

One afternoon in the hall, Paul Gertz told Pam that his son continued to do well; more than well, actually. Paul said he could see the pre-OS Daniel, the handsome young linebacker, emerging from the disease- and chemo-ravaged body Daniel had been occupying for the last year.

One thing that almost no one worried about anymore was Romy's heart. The threat of tachycardia had receded. Six months of chemotherapy had done nearly everything else to Romy: it had produced mouth sores, nausea, vomiting, PCP, baldness, lethargy, depression, and exhaustion, but not tachycardia. Romy's heart had stood up very well to Adriamycin, the most cardio-toxic drug in her treatment schedule. Or so it seemed. But on April 1, 1995, April Fool's Day, Romy's heart followed her knee and her lungs into revolt.

When Pam arrived in the room that morning, everything seemed normal. Romy was doing what she did every morning, watching *Gilligan's Island*. As the day progressed, she would also watch *The Jetsons*, Lucy and Ricky, Archie Bunker, Regis and Kathy Lee, *Geraldo*, and *Oprah*: a few weeks earlier, Pam had resolved that as soon as she did not have to worry anymore about Romy's dying, she was going to start worrying about Romy's TV habits.

Around eleven-fifteen, Kristin McCarthy, another favorite nurse, came into the room; Pam picked up a magazine and began to flip through it as Kristin removed a stethoscope from her pocket. A cardiac exam was part of the daily ward routine. Kristin placed the stethoscope on Romy's chest and listened for a moment.

"Do you feel okay, Rom?"

Pam put the magazine down. Eight months at NYU had made her an expert at reading voice inflections, and Kristin's voice suddenly sounded different. The girlish chumminess was gone; the young nurse sounded very cool and professional.

"Is everything all right, Kristin?" Pam asked.

Kristin ignored the question. "Do you feel okay, Rom?" she said again.

Romy nodded. "Uh-huh."

The bright red digital numbers on the cardiac monitor next to the bed were suddenly climbing: 130 . . . 140 beats per minute. . . . Pam's own heart began to race. . . . 150 . . . 160. The numbers on the monitor were changing nearly as quickly as the prices on a gas pump. At 250 beats per minute, the heart can go into flatline, stop completely.

Kristin left to find a resident.

"Does her heart always sound like this?" the young resident said to no one in particular. He moved the stethoscope to the right, then to the left, then up and down Romy's back. "You're sure you don't feel anything? No fluttery sensations or anything?"

Romy shook her head.

"Let's do an EKG," the resident said.

... 170 ... 180 ... 190 ... : As two orderlies wheeled an electrocardiograph into the room, the numbers on the cardiac monitor hit 200 beats per minute.

After the EKG was completed, the room emptied out again, except for Kristin, who remained standing in front of the monitor. Pam walked up behind her and peered over her shoulder. Romy's heartbeat was still climbing: 210 ... 220 ... 230....

"Kristin!" Pam almost shouted.

Just then, Dr. Paul MacGregor, an associate of Dr. Rausen's, walked into the room. He had Romy's EKG in his hand. The lines on the strip were violent and jagged and tightly bunched.

Dr. MacGregor smiled at Romy. "How are you feeling this morning, young lady?"

Romy shrugged. "Fine. A little tired maybe."

"No fluttery sensations?"

"Uh-uh."

"Good." Dr. MacGregor smiled. "Mrs. Hochman, could I have a word with you?"

"We're going to take her into the ICU," Dr. MacGregor said as soon as he and Pam were in the hall. "I don't think we ought to tell her; any agitation will only push the heartbeat higher. We don't want that now."

"So I shouldn't tell her she's going into the ICU?"

"No," Dr. MacGregor said.

Romy's heartbeat seemed to have stabilized. It was fluctuating between 230 and 240 when Pam returned to the room. A resident appeared in the doorway, then Kristin and another nurse; the second nurse was pushing a gurney. Romy looked alarmed. "Mom, where am I going?"

"I don't know, hon," Pam lied.

"You're just going for a little ride," Dr. MacGregor said.

A few seconds later, a flying wedge—Dr. MacGregor, Kristin, Pam, Romy, the other nurse, and the resident pushing the cardiac monitor—emerged from Romy's room at a half jog. The flying wedge made an abrupt right, Romy looked up. The ICU was a hundred feet away at the end of the hall. *"Mom! MOM!"*

Pam did not have the heart to lie again. "We're going to the ICU," Pam said, then immediately regretted it. The digital numbers on the cardiac machine jumped to 250.

Oh my God! I'm going to kill her, Pam thought. I'm going to kill my own child!

A week later, Romy was lying on an operating table looking up at the interior of her femoral artery. SONY, the logo on the television monitor said. The Hochmans used to have a Sony, Romy remembered, but the Sony above her head was much bigger. The monitor had a twenty-eight-, maybe a thirty-two-inch screen.

A tingling sensation—Romy squirmed. Was the metal snake moving? Dr. O'Connor had promised that the drugs would knock her out, but here she was, wide-awake. Romy looked up at the monitor. The snake was moving now, threading its way up through her body. In another minute or two, it would reach her heart.

Pam's blond head suddenly bobbed up. She was standing inside a glass booth on the other side of the room. Now a male head appeared: Dr. Brian O'Connor. Officially, Dr. O'Connor was known as a cardiac electrophysiologist, but he was really a kind of cardiac electrician. The beat of the human heart, like the hum of an air conditioner or hair dryer, is governed by electrical currents. Dr. O'Connor diagnosed and corrected current irregularities. A few days after the tachycardia episode, he told Pam and Jack that Romy's heart had two irregularities. "That's why the heart went into spasm," he said.

Jack asked if the irregularities could be corrected.

"Yes," the cardiologist said. "They can be burned out."

That was the task of the snake threading its way up through Romy's body. Once the pin-sized camera at the snake's head located the site of the irregularities on the surface of the cardiac muscle, Dr. O'Connor would maneuver the rest of the coil into position and administer a jolt of electricity. Called an ablation, the procedure is a form of electrocution; the portion of the heart muscle responsible for the current irregularity is quite literally burned to death.

Patients who have undergone the procedure—an individual must be awake when the electrical jolt is administered—describe the burning sensation produced by the jolt as unimaginably painful. Romy looked up at the monitor again. Her heart was coming into view now. There was the . . . the right atrium. She recognized it from eighth-grade biology. The snake was only an inch or so away from the site of the first irregularity. Drugs were supposed to sedate Romy until the ablation, but she still felt wide-awake. Someone was tugging at her shoulder. She looked up. Gail Garrity, one of her favorite nurses, was standing over her.

Gail smiled and said, "Dr. O'Connor's ready now." Groggily, Romy sat up. Abruptly, her head snapped back, then her entire body began to shake. Convulsions.

Inside the booth, Pam winced, then turned away.

"Got it," Dr. O'Connor said. There was excitement in his voice.

When Pam looked up again, Romy was lying on the table as limp as a Raggedy Ann doll. Pam shivered and turned away a second time.

"Here's the second irregularity."

A pouch-shaped object was expanding and contracting rhythmically on the monitor in front of Dr. O'Connor. The cardiologist bent forward and examined the image, then turned to Pam. "There's a difficulty," he said. "Here's where the heart's electrical impulses are located." He pointed a finger at a bundle of neurons near the top of the pouch-shaped object. "And here's the other irregularity." The cardiologist's finger barely moved. Only about a tenth of an inch separated the bundle from the site of the second malfunction.

Dr. O'Connor said he thought he could destroy the second site safely. But the margin was very narrow; the ablation could destroy a part of the heart wall. "There's a ten percent chance Romy could have a heart attack," he said. "I think we can avoid collateral damage." But there was a risk. He looked at Pam. "What do you want to do, Mrs. Hochman?"

For a moment, Pam thought the cardiologist was joking. No one had to make this kind of choice. Not in real life. This kind of thing only happened in books, books and nightmares.

"Mrs. Hochman?"

Pam looked out into the operating room. "Ten percent," she said.

"Romy could have another tach episode if we stop now," the doctor said.

Pam closed her eyes again. "All right, go ahead."

A moment later, she felt a hand on her arm. When she opened her eyes, Dr. O'Connor was smiling at her. "We're okay," he said. "I got it."

"No collateral damage?"

"No collateral damage."

Pam whispered a prayer of thanks.

A few weeks after the ablation, Romy made her one and only direct reference to the events of March 1995. It happened while the Hochmans were stuck in traffic on the FDR Drive. As soon as the car stopped, Romy's bald head emerged from the backseat. What was wrong? Why wasn't the car moving? Her voice was petulant, impatient.

Jack pointed at the cars around them. "Traffic jam. It'll clear up in a minute."

The bald head disappeared into the backseat again. Someone honked his horn. Someone else cursed, then suddenly, an angry voice exploded. "I don't want to be stuck. I don't want to be here. It's not fair, it's not fair! Everything happens to me! Why do I have to have all the bad luck? I hate it, I hate it."

This incident—or rather, its aftermath—also marked a milestone in Pam and Romy's relationship. For the first time in a very, very long time, Romy asked if she could sleep with Pam that night.

. . .

In April 1995, the rest of America was talking about the O. J. Simpson trial. But not the ninth floor—the ninth floor was talking about the only subject the ninth floor ever talks about: hope.

On nine, hope is perpetually debated, analyzed, deconstructed. There are also conversations about the deniers of hope; these are the doctors, who in the name of medical honesty insist on labeling terminally ill children terminally ill, thereby violating the floor's leading tenet about hope: every parent, most especially the parent of a dying child, has an inalienable right to the pursuit of hope.

A few parents remain impervious to the medical naysayers. They are the floor's fundamentalists, its radicals of hope, and in the spring of 1995, among the most radical of the radicals was Debbie Norberg. Debbie's hope was a natural wonder, like the Great Pyramids of Egypt or the Great Wall of China; it was an enormous black box a thousand miles long and a thousand miles high and utterly, utterly impenetrable. It allowed for no doubt, no uncertainty. It allowed for one thing and one thing only: Debbie's determination that her five-year-old Peter would not die, no matter what the doctors said.

In early March, this determination led to a disagreement between Debbie and Peter's oncologist, Dr. David Keough.* Debbie wanted Peter to have a bone marrow transplant; since NYU didn't do transplants, Dr. Keough had an easy way out. He could have just told her that the medical center didn't perform the procedure. Instead, he chose to tell Debbie that, in his opinion, a bone marrow transplant would only add needlessly to her son's already grievous suffering. Burkitt's lymphoma was a terminal condition.

"Basically, he wants me to take Peter home and let him die."

A few days after the conversation with Keough, Debbie and Pam were sitting in the courtyard, trying to warm themselves in a shaft of

*Pseudonym

early spring sunlight. A few feet away, two orderlies were arguing about the previous night's Bulls-Knicks game. Debbie took a puff of her cigarette. "I don't care what Keough says. I'm not going to give up."

Pam asked her what she intended to do.

"Find someone who will do a transplant. Wouldn't you, if it was Romy's only hope?"

Pam said yes, but after Debbie explained how a bone marrow transplant works, she was not so sure, not if Romy had Peter's prognosis. First, the marrow, the soft, pink-white substance at the center of the bone, is extracted via needles, very large needles; transplant needles are six to eight inches long. Next, chemotherapy at two, three, four times normal strength is pumped into the patient's body. Since the chemo wash obliterates disease-fighting white blood cells as well as cancer cells, next, the patient is isolated in a special infection-protected room. After his white blood cell count rises, the marrow is transfused back into his body.

In early April, over lunch at a coffee shop near NYU, Debbie told Pam that Memorial Sloan-Kettering had agreed to evaluate Peter for a transplant. "The doctors aren't making any promises," Debbie said. "But at least they are willing to consider Peter." She stopped suddenly and stared across the table. "Did you ever think that you'd be in a situation like this, ever?"

Pam shook her head. "Never."

"Part of me still believes I'm going to wake up any minute and say, 'See, I knew it; it was just a dream.' You ever feel that way?"

Pam said, "All the time."

"Keough's wrong," Debbie said. "I know he's wrong."

Pam did not think Keough was wrong. But she'd never tell Debbie that. She did not want to be the destroyer of hope.

CHAPTER TEN

OVER THE WINTER, ROMY HAD A CHANGE OF HEART ABOUT DR. Rausen. She wasn't ready to be president of the Aaron Rausen fan club or anything. But after she had stopped being angry at him she discovered that, in his own gruff, distracted way, Dr. Rausen could be wry, funny, even sweet. True, he never actually talked to you—like a lot of Great Men, he was more a monologuist than a conversationalist—but Romy didn't mind that; she was a natural listener. And Dr. Rausen was a very good storyteller.

One of his best stories was about Sergei from Brighton Beach. Sergei was so tough that even in summer he wore a long black leather trench coat. "You know what he did at the end of our first meeting?" Dr. Rausen said one day.

Romy said she had no idea.

"Sergei took five thousand dollars out of his jacket pocket, put it on the table and said, 'This is a down payment on my daughter's treatment.' " (Sergei's daughter had leukemia.) "You know what he took out next?" Dr. Rausen continued. "A knife. He told me if I didn't save his daughter, he would kill me."

"What did you do?" Romy asked.

The physician pointed out that he was from the old neighborhood. The Lower East Side. "It was a pretty tough place when I was growing up."

Dr. Rausen as a juvenile delinquent was even harder to imagine than Dr. Rausen wrestling a knife out of Sergei's hand. Romy asked him what he really did.

"I called security."

In September, Dr. Rausen had seemed like God himself, but little by little the monologues began to humanize him. One of Romy's favorite stories was about how he became a doctor. It was because of his younger brother Milton, Dr. Rausen said. One morning in 1943 five-year-old Milton Rausen woke up with a terrible headache. The next day, Milton was too sick to get out of bed. The day after that, Milton was rushed uptown to New York Hospital. Two weeks later, Milton was dead of spinal meningitis. "I only realized it later," Dr. Rausen said, "but I became a physician because I never wanted to see another child suffer the way Milton suffered."

After this story, Romy liked Dr. Rausen even more.

Chemotherapy impedes healing, and in April the cumulative effects of three months of postoperative chemo had made Romy's knee vulnerable to a new problem.

"Whoops, I think you have a little infection here," a nurse said one afternoon. Romy sat up in the bed and looked at her leg. A greenish-yellow fluid was oozing from the scab on top of the incision. The nurse finished cutting away the bandage, then probed the scab gently with a finger. Romy was surprised; the scab, rock-hard since January, moved. Pam arrived while the nurse was putting a fresh bandage on the knee.

"If I were you," the nurse said, "I'd have Pearlman look at the scab. It looks ready to fall off."

A few days later, Dr. Pearlman sent an associate, Lewis Goldenberg,* a specialist in surgical wounds, to perform the examination. After poking and probing at the scab for a few moments, Dr. Goldenberg pronounced the incision infected but not seriously. Neosporin and daily bandage changes would keep the infection under control until Romy finished chemotherapy in July, then a skin graft could be done. Doing a graft now would be pointless, Dr. Goldenberg said; nothing heals properly on chemo.

On May fifth, Romy's knee began to hurt again for the first time since October. "Do you want me to call Pearlman?" Pam asked. After a few minutes of debate, she and Romy decided to wait. Today was Friday. They would see what happened over the weekend. Infections were notoriously unpredictable. Maybe this one would clear up on its own.

At around two the next morning, Pam awoke to someone tugging at her T-shirt. Romy. "Terrible shooting pains," she gasped, "right here . . ." Romy pointed to her leg. At eight o'clock, Pam called Dr. Pearlman; his answering service said the doctor would be unavailable today. Pam cursed and looked over at Romy. She was lying on the bed with her eyes closed; her face was ashen and drawn; she had not slept at all that night.

"Is the pain any better, hon?"

Romy shook her head.

Dr. Rausen usually spent weekends at his country house in Westport, but Pam decided to call his apartment anyway. If there was any truth to the law of averages, they were due for some luck. The phone rang three times before a gravelly, liquid voice said hello. An emergency had kept Dr. Rausen in town Friday night. He was just about to leave his apartment for Connecticut when Pam phoned.

Percoset and Valium, the two drugs Dr. Rausen prescribed, brought

*Pseudonym

some relief, but Saturday evening the pain began to bore through the drug screen. On Sunday morning, Romy awoke to a knee that had swollen up completely. Now she looked as if she had two kneecaps again.

Dr. Rausen, now in Westport, ordered an ambulance to pick Romy up at Ronald McDonald House.

Romy, who can calibrate the quality of pain as expertly as an Eskimo can calibrate the quality of snow, says that no pain she experienced during her illness can match the pain she experienced that Sunday afternoon at the hands of the two ambulance drivers. The throbbing, swollen knee, sensitive to even a gentle touch, was banged, bumped, jarred, and jostled from bed to hall to lobby to ambulance. Immobilized on the gurney by two canvas belts, Romy remembers wondering why she was still awake; excruciating pain, she had read somewhere, was supposed to make you pass out.

On Sunday, Dr. Pearlman was back in New York. He ordered a new C/T scan and blood cultures of the incision. The next morning, when he returned with the results, Pam and Romy were having a fight.

Unable to control her health, her time, her diet, anything about her life, Romy had developed an obsessive Captain Queeg–like need to control the making of her bed. Everything—the sheets, the pillows, the spread—had to be done exactly right; otherwise, Romy would insist that the bed be remade. This morning's fight was over the top sheet: Romy was insisting it be folded back exactly six inches when Dr. Pearlman walked in.

The surgeon began on an upbeat note. Everything—the blood cultures, the scan, and the small amount of drainage in the incision—argued for a treatable minor infection. But midway through the conversation, the A word surfaced for the first time since January. Dr. Pearlman said he might have to amputate if the infection persisted. But Romy, an experienced Pearlmanologist, was not alarmed; Pearlman loved to tell you the absolute worst thing that could happen to you.

"I'm going to put her on a new antibiotic regimen today," the surgeon told Pam as he was leaving. "Let's see how the knee responds."

A week later, the knee was deemed well enough to allow its owner to take it to Ronald McDonald House for the Mother's Day weekend.

On Sunday morning, Pam received a pair of earrings and a card. The card read:

I want to thank you for being here for me. You're the best mother in the whole world.

Love,
Romy

Pam also had a present for Romy: two airline tickets to Los Angeles.

Romy's last chemotherapy treatment, a twelve-hour methotrexate drip, was scheduled for July 20; American Airlines flight 19 left Kennedy Airport three days later, July 23, at 10:30 A.M. California was so close now, Romy could almost feel the sun on her face.

As Pam was going to bed that night, Debbie Norberg called. She said she was bringing Peter home from Sloan-Kettering on Wednesday; the bone marrow transplant had failed. "Some Mother's Day present, huh?" Debbie said, and hung up.

In mid-June, during a visit to Pam's parents' house on Cape Cod, the infection in the knee flared up again.

"You think the incision's draining again?" Pam asked.

"I think it's swollen again, too." Romy still had sleep in her eyes. As soon as she woke up, she had hobbled out to the front porch in search of Pam.

Gently, Pam picked up Romy's leg, put it on her lap and pushed the flannel nightie back to the thigh. Romy was right. Overnight a dark stain had formed in the middle of the bandage. There was renewed swelling too. Except now the swelling extended to the area below the knee. "The infection is back, Rom." Gently, Pam lowered the leg to the floor and went inside to call Dr. Pearlman.

Monday afternoon, after inspecting her knee, Dr. Pearlman announced that the evidence—a new C/T scan and blood cultures—still pointed to a superficial infection. Deep infections, infections involving the bone, produce great globs of mucousy pus, he said. Romy's knee was just oozing a little.

"I know that," Pam said.

"Well, that's good. We should feel happy about that."

"I'll feel happy when the knee heals. When's that going to happen, Doctor?"

Dr. Pearlman said what was needed was a month without chemo. He was going to ask Dr. Rausen to postpone Romy's last treatment for a month, from July 20 to August 20. Minus immune-suppressing methotrexate, the antibiotics might be able to snuff out the infection for good. The trip to California would have to be postponed.

When Pam asked what would happen if the drugs failed, Dr. Pearlman repeated the scenario he had outlined in May: Replace the prosthesis with a plastic spacer, and if that failed, probably amputation. In the edited version of this conversation Romy got, the surgeon's second option was translated into an innocuous "We'll see." If the bone turned out to be infected, Pam said, Dr. Pearlman would remove the prosthesis, and if that option failed, "Well, we'll see," Pam said.

However, Pearlmanolgist Romy knew what "we'll see" meant. "That means he might amputate, right?"

"Dr. Pearlman said it can't be ruled out, Rom."

When Pam went down to the cafeteria, Romy closed her eyes and tried to imagine what life would be like with one leg. Sports would be out, but she had never been much of an athlete anyway. Boys . . . boys would definitely be a problem, but she could not have children anyway. The beach . . . there would be no getting around the beach. She would always have to wear long pants to the beach. But amputation also offered compensations, the biggest being that she would finally be rid of the hateful knee. Her leg, Romy would miss, but her knee, never. The knee had betrayed her, lied to her, abused her, almost killed her. What's more, even rehabilitated, the knee would still be a cheat. It would only provide a 35-degree range of motion, the same range as a leg prosthesis. Whether the knee stayed or went, Romy would still walk with a limp for the rest of her life.

When Pam came back, Romy said she did not think amputation such a terrible option. She could walk just as well on a leg prosthesis, and her awful knee would be gone for good.

"We'll see," Pam said quietly.

The next morning, Pam dropped by her lawyer's office to sign Jack's going-away present to her, a joint custody agreement. Then she borrowed his car and drove over to Staten Island to visit Debbie Norberg. Debbie, fierce, ever-believing Debbie, had stopped believing. Peter was going to die; all Debbie could do now was sit in this little two-story house across from Sal's Pizzeria and bear witness, bear witness and try not to go crazy.

A thick medicinal odor intermingled with food smells in the small Norberg apartment. Pam was not sure where the odor was coming from until Debbie led her into a room off the kitchen: Peter's room. He was asleep on the bed. Pam walked over and looked at him. His face, swollen to almost twice its normal size, looked absurd on his little-boy body; it was like the beach-ball heads children draw on stick figures. A thick, mucousy substance was oozing from his eyes. Pam could only look for a moment.

She turned to Debbie. "Is he having trouble seeing?"

"Uh-huh—the swelling." Debbie bent down and stroked a sweaty, flushed cheek.

One eye opened. The flesh around it was so swollen, Pam could barely see the eyeball.

"Oh, come on, baby." A half hour later, Debbie, camera in hand, was trying to get Peter to pose for a picture with Pam.

"No, no," he said angrily. "I don't wanna have my picture taken."

Debbie handed the camera to Peter. "Okay, Mr. Cranky Pants, take a picture of me and Pam, then."

Peter grumpily acceded to this suggestion. But Pam's praise of his Polaroid—about what you would expect from a five-year-old, two pairs of legs and a large expanse of floor—only produced more anger. He told Pam, "I hate the picture and I hate you."

Pam knew there was a logical explanation for the anger: the painkillers. Painkillers made Peter mad at everyone—at his mother, the doctors, the nurses, at the world. She had seen it happen a half dozen times before. Still, Pam couldn't help wondering.

Cognitive psychologists say only a youngster about Lotte Kauffman's age—sixteen—is able to feel a sense of injustice, a sense of being terribly wronged. But perhaps, Pam thought, the imminence of death makes a child precocious.

Three and a half weeks later, at 8 A.M. on the morning of July 29, five-year-old Peter died in his own home and in his mother's arms. His death was very peaceful, Debbie said a few days later. "We were lying on the living room couch together; Peter opened his eyes a little, and looked at me. Then he just stopped breathing." Debbie paused for a moment, then said, "I saw him take his first breath, Pam . . . and I saw him take his last."

In August, Romy came full circle. On the tenth, she and Pam drove down to Rehoboth Beach, in Delaware, for the Hochmans' annual summer reunion. Romy, always excited to be in Rehoboth, was especially excited this year. The Katz-Lewises were flying in from San Francisco next week and she would meet them in a new wardrobe, a California wardrobe. George Hochman had promised to give her a thousand dollars to buy new clothes.

On the twelfth, Amy, armed with George's American Express card, was supposed to take Romy on a shopping spree. But then, as usual, everything that could go wrong, did.

On the eleventh, Amy was suddenly called back to Washington on a work emergency. Then George Hochman refused to give Pam his AmEx card so she could buy the clothes for Romy.

"But, Dad," Amy pleaded before she left, "this isn't for Pam, it's for Romy."

"No," George said. In Smithtown, Pam had used credit cards like an automatic weapon. Trusting her with a credit card would be crazy. The shopping spree was postponed until Aunt Amy was available.

The next day, the knee, apparently restless and bored with beach life, flared up again. On the morning of the thirteenth, Romy awoke to two familiar symptoms, pain and swelling, and one new one: weltlike bumps. There was also another ominous change; drainage from the surgical incision, previously minimal, now became significant.

"Don't deep infections drain a lot?" Romy said when she showed Pam the stained bandage.

"According to Pearlman . . ." Pam said. "I'm going to call him."

But Dr. Pearlman was on vacation, too. Pam called Dr. Rausen. Two hours later, his associate Paul MacGregor ordered the Hochmans back to New York. The next day, a small globule of pus was drained from one of the new bumps on the knee and sent down to a laboratory on the fourth floor for analysis.

Dr. MacGregor, who had rescued Romy in March, rescued her again now. This lab test, perhaps the seventh or eighth done on the wound, finally produced a definitive diagnosis. The proximal tibia bone was infected; a microbe called *Staphylococcus aureus* had set up house there. Since the bone was involved, technically, Romy had a deep infection. But Dr. MacGregor said that the *S. aureus* microbe is very vulnerable to antibiotics.

The Hochmans were now due to leave for Los Angeles on September 11. Pam asked if she should reschedule the flight.

Dr. MacGregor smiled and said, "They have drugstores in Los Angeles, don't they?"

On Wednesday, August 22, after her final methotrexate treatment, Pam took Romy down to the radiology department for a final scan. It was late afternoon and the reception area was empty except for a shaft of afternoon sunlight and a single patient, a young man in a wheelchair. He turned around when Pam and Romy arrived.

Daniel Gertz.

Daniel's latest lung scan had come back positive; there were five black spots on it. The largest spot was no bigger than a small pinprick, the smallest so small that the unaided eye could barely see it. Tiny as they were, the spots were full of meaning. At a minimum, they meant Daniel would have to go through the whole awful treatment process again: surgery (to remove the growths in the lungs), chemotherapy, nausea, vomiting, baldness—all of it. The spots also meant that what the Gertz family had been through so far was nothing compared to what they were about to go through.

The CCG computer in Arcadia, California, now had treatment outcomes on all four of the 0133 subjects Romy knew about. Somewhere in its database Daniel, Lotte Kauffman, and Justin Gitlin were listed as Arm B treatment failures and Moira Blake, who was in the same treatment group as Romy, as an Arm D failure.

Daniel, aware of his talisman's role for Romy, seemed to feel that he had let her down by relapsing. "You know," he said, "just because this happened to me doesn't mean it's going to happen to you. You're going to do fine, I know you are. No one with a 100 percent count ever comes back."

A technician emerged from a scan room. "Romy Hochman."

Pam put her hand on Daniel's wheelchair. "I don't want to leave you here by yourself."

Daniel said Paul would be back in a minute. He was making a call in the hall.

As the technicians were preparing to slide her into the C/T

machine, Romy asked Pam to hold her ankle while she was inside. She had never done that before.

That night, Romy described the encounter with Daniel in a letter to her aunt Amy.

Dear Amy:

Today was an awful day. While I was down in radiology I saw Daniel Gertz. He was in a hospital robe and had an IV. At first I didn't even think it was him. It ended up that he had a recurrence.

I'm kinda scared now. I mean, while everyone kept coming back, I always held on to Daniel as the "ok" one. Now he's back and I have no one to hold on to as "ok." I guess I just have to hold on to the one hundred percent thing. But it's still hard. I'd rather have a person to hold on to than a number.

Love,
Romy

Ninth-floor rules say that, once discharged, a patient is never supposed to voluntarily return to the floor. But on September 2, Romy decided to risk the wrath of nine's gods and say a final good-bye to the three nurses who had befriended her over the past year: Kelly Cervone, Gail Garrity, and Vicki Vecorello. Later in the week, she made a final visit to Dr. Rausen's office on East Thirty-fourth Street, where she was the recipient of a gruff good-bye and an even gruffer hug. On her way out of the office, Romy paused briefly at the doorway to the conference room and looked in. It had been almost eleven months to the day since she had been officially designated a cancer patient in this room.

September 10, Romy's last full day in New York, was passed quietly: lunch with her father at Zillini's, an Italian restaurant on the corner of Seventy-third and First Avenue near Ronald McDonald House, some clothes shopping at Saks in the afternoon, and a movie that night. · She and her mother rented *Sleepless in Seattle* again.

Pam's year in New York ended more dramatically: a papal mass in Central Park. On the Friday before the mass, Debbie called and said she had an extra ticket. "I know you've got a lot of packing to do and everything, but I thought maybe you might want to come with me."

Pam knew the remark about packing was code for "I know you're not a Catholic."

"I'd love to come," she said. "Sunday morning?"

"On the Great Lawn in Central Park," Debbie said. "I'll pick you up at seven-thirty."

Sunday morning was a perfect September morning, cool and clear and golden. Pam and Debbie arrived an hour early. But the Great Lawn was already full; a crowd of 200,000 or 300,000 people was spread out in all directions from a giant screen set on a stage in the center of the lawn. Pam had never seen so many people in one place before. But the crowd was remarkably calm, almost serene. No one was talking loudly, or jostling, or pushing, or shoving.

Near the southern edge of the lawn, there was an empty spot in a grove of trees; Pam and Debbie walked over and sat down. The stage where the pope was to say mass was several hundred feet away. But the enormous TV monitor would make every papal movement and facial gesture visible for miles. When it came to life a few minutes later, Pam was surprised; the man on the screen was very different from the stooped, elderly figure she had seen in photos. He was broad-shouldered and powerful-looking and he had a wonderful face: kind and strong and pure and, above all, still.

Looking at the face, Pam felt the pain of the past year begin to drain away. They were going to be all right now, she was certain . . . she and Romy. They had won . . . the war was over, and they had survived . . . both of them.

At the end of the mass, cages next to the stage sprang open and the crisp autumn blue sky above the Great Lawn filled with hundreds of white doves. Debbie looked up and pointed.

"There's my baby, there's my Peter."

There were so many doves in the sky, Pam couldn't tell which one Debbie was pointing at.

"Do you see him? Do you see him?" Debbie was shouting now.

"Yes, yes, I see him," Pam lied.

"Good-bye, Peter," Debbie whispered. "Good-bye, my precious baby."

As John Paul pronounced a final benediction, Pam said a prayer of her own, a prayer for Peter, for Lotte, for Jimmy Moriarty, and for all the other children who had left the ninth floor.

JULIE AND HER SISTERS

CHAPTER ONE

THERE IS A MARY POPPINS BOOK IN JULIE'S EARLIEST MEMORY; SO SHE dates the memory to 1964, the year the Disney movie appeared and the year she turned four. The memory also has October light in it, so the incident Julie is recalling must have occurred in the autumn of that year. The light streams through the venetian blinds over the couch and onto the living-room rug, where it makes a grillwork pattern of gold bars on the cover of the Mary Poppins book.

Julie and her mother are sitting on the couch watching *One Life to Live*. Kay Mackey watches *One Life* every afternoon. Julie likes to watch it, too.

The warm fall sunlight, and the rhythmic up and down of the perfectly modulated television voices make Julie drowsy. She is just about to fall asleep when someone bangs on the door.

Her mother stiffens. "The kitchen door must be locked," Kay says, "I better let them in."

Julie knows who "them" is: Jennifer and Susan, her noisy, bickering big sisters. Jennifer and Susan are home from school already. Julie, who cannot conceive of a more perfect moment than this, pleads with her mother to stay.

Kay pretends to be shocked. "Julie," she says. "Do you want your sisters to stand on the back porch all afternoon?"

Julie would not mind, but she knows that if she says so, she will be scolded.

There is a strange odor in Julie's next memory. A hospital odor, the smell of alcohol and disinfectant. This memory can be dated with absolute accuracy: the morning of July 17, 1967, her mother's thirty-seventh birthday. Big sisters Jennifer and Susan are also in this memory. Everyone is except little Lisa and Emily. This morning Julie's father, Bob, said that the baby sisters were too young to go to the hospital. Grandmother Eunice, Kay's mother, is coming over soon to sit for them. Julie almost feels sorry for Lisa and Emily, but, then, if everyone went to the hospital, going to the hospital would not be such a great honor.

The older Mackey children are quiet on the drive to the hospital. Julie's big brother, Bob Junior, almost thirteen now, asks his father a question about a baseball player, then opens the comic book in his lap. Jennifer, the next oldest sibling, does not speak at all. She stares out the window all the way from Huntingdon Valley, where the Mackeys live, to downtown Philadelphia. Julie is puzzled by the quiet. Usually, her older brother and sister are very chatty on family drives. Bob makes silly jokes, and Jennifer, who knows everything but is bossy, orders the younger sisters around.

At the hospital entrance, Julie asks her brother, Bob, where they are. "Jefferson Hospital," he says.

A nurse has to help Kay into the waiting room. This worries Julie. So does her mother's appearance. Kay looks thinner than Julie remembers, thinner and frailer, but when Kay smiles Julie feels better. She looks around: Jennifer and Susan and Bob Junior are smiling too.

"Okay, kids, ready?" Julie's father, Bob, says. Julie gets up and joins Susan and Jennifer and Bob Junior, who are lined up in front of a waiting-room window. The four children begin to sing "Happy Birthday." The song was Jennifer's idea; she suggested it this morning at breakfast. In addition to being bossy and knowing everything, Jennifer thinks of everything, too. Julie has heard the adults say that without Jennifer, Bob Senior could not get by in this terrible time. Jennifer is a godsend; only nine but already a little woman.

The song goes well for a chorus, but then everyone starts to cry. Julie is not immediately distressed when Kay bursts into tears or when Jennifer and Susan do; sometimes mothers and sisters cry. But Julie is tremendously worried by the tears of her father and brother. In her experience, big brothers and fathers never cry—at least, they never cry under any circumstances Julie's young mind can conceive.

Only the sisters are in Julie's next memory.

Jennifer, Susan, Lisa, and Julie herself; the four of them are kneeling in prayer beside her grandmother's four-poster bed. It is a steamy August afternoon a month after Kay's birthday party, and Grandmother Eunice has just come into the bedroom and said that Kay is dead. Julie still remembers exactly how her grandmother told them.

"Girls," she said, "your father has just called me from the hospital. He says your mother is in heaven now. You don't have to cry. Heaven is a good place. Your mother will be happy there. She will be able to watch down on all of you and she won't be in pain. There is no pain in heaven."

Julie Mackey Conte was born on November 12, 1960, at St. Bonaventure Hospital in Philadelphia and grew up in Huntingdon Valley, a middle-class suburb of the city. Julie describes the Huntingdon Valley of her childhood as Leave It to Beaver Land; there were working fathers and stay-at-home mothers, green lawns and unlocked doors, backyard barbecues and streets full of footloose children. Like the Mackeys, everyone else in town was Catholic, Italian or Irish (Julie is a little of both), and nearly everyone had a big family, though even in Huntingdon

Valley, few families were as big as Julie's. Roughly every eighteen months between 1956 and 1964, Bob, a court stenographer, and Kay Mackey, a former law clerk, had a child: first, Bob Junior, then Jennifer, Susan, Julie, Lisa, and finally, in early 1965, Emily.

Julie says that after Emily's birth everything changed. Six months later, Kay was diagnosed with breast cancer. In August, she had a mastectomy at Jefferson Hospital. A course of radiation (in the mid-1960s, chemotherapy was not routinely used against breast cancer) followed; then Kay returned to Huntingdon Valley. A year later she was sick again—agonizing bone pain this time. "Relapse," said the doctors at Jefferson Hospital. Two months later, Julie and Jennifer helped Kay take down the storm windows. Six months after that, Kay was dead.

Second sister Susan, who was ten when her mother died, says that of all the sisters, Julie most resembles pretty, sweet-tempered, dark-haired, blue-eyed Kay. Susan recalls that for Julie's first Halloween in the house that she and husband Peter moved into as newlyweds, Julie made pumpkin cutouts and an elaborate Casper the Friendly Ghost for the front porch. "That's the kind of thing my mother used to do," Susan declares.

The Mackey sisters have one-word designations for each other. Susan says she is known as the quiet sister, Emily is the organized sister, Lisa the spunky sister, Jennifer the leader sister. Julie, she says, is the nice sister.

Julie, however, is ambivalent about her designation. Sometimes she thinks that she is too nice for her own good.

It is 1972 now, and Julie, twelve, is rummaging through a bureau in Jennifer's bedroom. Underneath a pile of sweaters she feels something crumply, papery. A newspaper clipping. The clipping is brown and frayed with age. Julie pulls it out and reads the headline. KAY MACKEY

DIES AT 37. Her mother's obituary notice. Julie is not surprised to find it hidden. Kay is almost a nonperson in the house now; the sisters speak about her, but only among themselves. At the bottom of the obituary, next to a not-very-good photo, Kay's cause of death is listed as breast cancer.

Julie feels no sense of personal resonance when she reads this. The obituary is sad, losing her mother was sad, but breast cancer, the disease that killed Kay, feels as remote to twelve-year-old Julie as a flood in China or an earthquake in Chile.

Julie slips the clipping back under the sweaters so Yvonne won't see it. Yvonne is the sisters' new stepmother; since her marriage to Bob Senior in 1969, all personal mementos and photos of Kay have disappeared; they are all packed away in the basement now. A division also has developed within the family. The sisters and older brother, Bob, have pulled away from Yvonne and their father and formed their own separate family with Jennifer, the oldest sister, as its head.

Today, the other sisters speak of Jennifer not as a big sister, but as a beloved parent. It was Jennifer who told Julie what would happen when she got her period, who showed ten-year-old Emily how to comb the kinks out of her hair, and taught thirteen-year-old Susan to apply lipstick.

It is 1979 now, early September, and Julie is at her bedroom door. Lisa is standing behind her. Downstairs in the living room, Jennifer and her father are shouting at each other. Their voices are too chaotic to be intelligible. But Julie and Lisa know what the fight is about. Jennifer has just returned from a summer in Arizona. The trip was made against her father's and Yvonne's wishes. All summer the other sisters have wondered what would happen when Jennifer returned.

Suddenly, the shouting subsides. There are only murmurs now. Someone taps on the bedroom door. Julie opens it slightly. It's Susan. "I think it's going to be okay," Susan whispers. "I've been spying. I think they're going to be able to talk it out."

A few minutes later, the front door opens. Everyone recognizes the footsteps. Yvonne is home. The shouting begins again; this time it is louder, more violent. Someone begins to cry; Jennifer, yes, definitely

Jennifer. More steps. Jennifer's this time. There is more shouting. The front door opens. Someone is leaving. The door slams shut and all at once it is quiet downstairs.

After this night, the sisters do not see Jennifer again for seven years.

In 1987, when she was twenty-seven, Julie met a young man named Peter Conte on a blind date. Peter, an electrical engineer, was a year older and worked for a large computer company. Julie liked him immediately. "I had seen enough of the bad stuff to recognize the good stuff when I saw it," she says. Peter had dark, liquid eyes, a shy, self-effacing sense of humor, and understated good looks. Peter was like her, Julie thought, practical, down-to-earth, a no-frills person.

One day, about four or five weeks after they met—Julie thinks it might have been mid-October, because there were Halloween decorations in the store windows—she and Peter ran into her aunt Grace outside a department store in Philadelphia. Later, walking to the garage where they had parked, Peter asked about the family connection. He was intrigued by Grace; she was grand, imposing, an Auntie Mame–ish sort of woman, very unlike Julie.

"Her husband's sort of a big deal," Julie said. "He's the executive vice president . . ." Julie mentioned the name of a large steel company, then, without quite intending to, she began to tell Peter about her mother, about how Kay had died young of breast cancer. They were in the garage next to Peter's car by the time Julie finished her story.

"How old were you when your mother died?" Peter asked.

"Five and a half," Julie said.

Neither of them spoke for a moment, then Peter said, "You were young."

"Yes," Julie said. "Very."

According to Peter, this talk did not make any special impression on him. For a long time, he says, Julie's family history and the facts of her mother's death just seemed to be incidental biographical detail. He knew that Julie had grown up in Huntingdon Valley, had a wealthy aunt named Grace, four sisters, and a brother, a degree in biology from Villanova, blue eyes, frizzy dark hair, a wonderful smile, and a mother who died young of breast cancer. Not until later did any one fact seem more or less important than any other.

In September 1988, Peter and Julie were married at Don Bosco Church in Hapsboro, Pennsylvania. Susan was the maid of honor, younger sisters Emily and Lisa the bridesmaids. But Jennifer, the "first" sister, the sister everybody else looked up to, was absent.

Julie and Jennifer had decided that in the interest of family harmony, Jennifer should remain in Phoenix, where she lived with her husband, Rick. Her father and Yvonne still had not forgiven Jennifer for making that trip to Arizona and for moving there for good in the fall of 1979, after the fight.

In 1990, when Jennifer announced that she was pregnant, the other sisters were thrilled. But they were worried, too. How could they not be? The last time a Mackey woman bore a child, she lost her breast and then her life. But this collective spasm of sisterly anxiety subsided quickly. Jennifer was a healthy, vital young woman. When you looked at the situation rationally, the sisters told themselves, what was there to worry about?

Lisa, the spunky sister, is also the most fatalistic. Growing up, Lisa would occasionally be visited by an awful fear: None of the sisters would ever live to see their children come of age. But Jennifer's normal pregnancy, which produced a daughter, Deidre, made even Lisa stop worrying. What happened to their mother was not a curse or a sign of cosmic displeasure after all. It was just a fluke.

One night in February 1992, Jennifer called the sisters to announce that she was pregnant again. Within six months, Julie and Lisa were also pregnant.

A certain amount of breast discomfort is normal in pregnancy, so in June 1992, when Jennifer began to complain about an aching breast, Julie was not immediately alarmed. Her own breasts were already beginning to feel sensitive, and Jennifer was five months further into her pregnancy. But in mid-July, Jennifer said the ache was unusual; it did not feel like the normal soreness and discomfort of a pregnant woman's breast.

Three weeks later, the ache became a pain. The first time Julie heard Jennifer use the word "pain," she felt a flutter of anxiety, like the beating of butterfly wings against the inside of her chest. It was not like Jennifer—not like any of the sisters—to complain, not unless something really hurt. Jennifer said that there were no physical changes; her left breast looked and felt perfectly normal. She and her obstetrician had both palpated it. It felt like a big, fat, pregnant woman's breast.

"Do you think Jennifer's obstetrician knows about Mom?" Julie asked Peter the next day.

Their mother also had breast pain during her last pregnancy, and she was the same age—thirty-four—as Jennifer.

"I'm sure she does," Peter said.

Jennifer gave birth to her second daughter, Melody, in mid-October. The delivery was uneventful, but the mammogram that followed the delivery was not. "There is nothing to worry about," Jennifer said when she called Julie in early November to report that a tumor had been found on her mammogram. "They got it early and the tumor is very small," Jennifer said. "I have a great prognosis."

After Julie hung up, she and Peter talked for a while, then he went into the living room and turned on the television. Jennifer was not mentioned again until the Contes were in bed. Julie was almost asleep when she heard a rustling sound; she opened her eyes. Peter was propped up in the bed beside her.

"Could it happen to you?" he said. "What happened to Jennifer?"

Julie had considered the question before, of course, but never in this context. She stared into the dark for a moment, then said, "Yes, it could happen to me."

CHAPTER TWO

LISA HAD BEEN EXPECTING THE CALL FOR AS LONG AS SHE COULD remember. But in her imaginings, it always arrived accompanied by thunderbolts and wailing cherubim. Real life, as usual, proved less imaginative. The evening Jennifer called, Lisa was standing by the stove with an overdue cable bill in her hand listening to the theme music from *Jeopardy* drift in from the living-room TV.

"I'm fine. Don't worry, they caught it in time," Jennifer said very quickly.

For a moment, Lisa felt disoriented; it was not supposed to happen this way. Alex Trebek was not supposed to be talking in the background and Julie was supposed to be on the phone. Lisa was sure that Julie would be the first to call; she was the sister who bruised easiest, wasn't she?

"Can Andy do anything to help?" Lisa asked. Her husband, Andrew Di Salvo, was a physician.

"No—and please tell Andy not to worry."

There was a pause, then Jennifer said she was having a mastectomy on December 12. "Emily is coming down on the tenth; she's going to help out. Rick and the kids are really looking forward to the visit. You're going to be okay with this now, aren't you, Lisa? I'm counting on you."

Jennifer's voice was suddenly very businesslike. Lisa imagined that this was the voice Jennifer the stockbroker used when her clients called all frantic and panicky and wanting to sell when the Dow took a dip.

"Uh-huh, I'm all right," Lisa said. There was something wet on her face, right below her eyes. Tears.

"Promise me you won't worry. C'mon, I want to hear it."

"I promise," Lisa said. She took a deep breath. Her eyes were very wet now.

"You're sure?" Jennifer said.

"I'm sure."

Lisa maintained her composure until Jennifer hung up, then she slumped against the refrigerator door and began to sob.

She was still crying when Andy walked into the kitchen a few minutes later. He put his arms around her and asked what was wrong. Lisa tried to tell him, but she kept stopping on the word "Jennifer." It was like a giant unscalable wall in her mind; every time Lisa said "Jennifer," she burst into tears again.

On December 12, Jennifer's left breast and one small pearl-shaped lymph node adjacent to the breast were removed at a Phoenix hospital. "The surgeon got it all," Jennifer announced the next day in a round of phone calls to Pennsylvania. "I'm going to be fine." Eight weeks later, Julie gave birth to her first child, Brittany. Lisa's first child, Andy ("little Andy"), was born four months later.

Jennifer looked sensational when she flew east in June for her brother Bob's wedding. She was slim and blond and tan from the Arizona sun. No one could remember her looking better.

"Have you ever seen a mastectomy scar?" Jennifer asked Emily the morning of the wedding. The two sisters were getting dressed in Aunt Grace's bedroom.

Emily had, actually, seen a recent PBS medical documentary that had included a scene of a Japanese surgeon holding a newly removed breast; he was showing it to the patient's family—to her husband and mother and sister. The breast looked like a small, freshly severed head. Emily was so appalled by the oozing liquid flesh in the surgeon's hand that she had to turn away from the screen.

No, Emily lied now, she never had.

Jennifer opened her robe.

No traces of violence, no long, ugly scar. Just a neat little incision about six inches long on the left side of Jennifer's chest.

"Do you want to touch it?" Jennifer asked.

Emily was not sure she did, but how could she refuse? Jennifer, private even with the other sisters, was offering an incredible intimacy. Emily looked at the scar again. It was shaped like a half-moon.

Jennifer must have sensed her nervousness. She took Emily's hand and ran it across the incision. The surface of the scar felt nubby and grainy.

Jennifer smiled and closed her robe. "Not so bad, is it?"

Emily smiled back. "No, not at all."

A few days after Jennifer flew home, Emily told Julie that she wasn't going to worry anymore; Jennifer was going to make a complete recovery. Julie said she felt confident too. But in late October, Julie felt another flutter of butterfly wings against her chest. During a phone conversation, Jennifer complained of hip discomfort.

"No, it's not *that*," she said when Julie asked if anything else was bothering her. "I think it's because of the new van." The door on her van was set very high, Jennifer explained. "Getting in and out with the baby . . . I think I must have pulled something."

But at the end of November, Jennifer complained about her hip again. "Rick and I have traded cars," she said one night. "I'm driving the Accord now. It's easier to get into than the van."

Julie was surprised. "Does your hip hurt you that much?" she asked.

"When I raise my leg it does."

Jennifer also had a dry cough. But the cough was from the flu, Jennifer was sure of it. "Everyone out here has a bug," she told Julie.

"When was the last time you saw your oncologist?" Julie asked.

"In October . . ." Jennifer said. "The beginning of October. I get checked every three months. If there was anything funny, they'd see it. I'm not worried, and you shouldn't be either."

Julie said she was not worried. But when she hung up, she realized that she had forgotten to tell Jennifer that she was pregnant again.

Jennifer's next exam was on January 5. Julie was washing the dinner dishes when Jennifer called on the evening of the sixth.

"Relapse," Jennifer said. ". . . Spread to the bones . . . doctors optimistic . . . I feel fine . . . Don't worry." Before Julie had a chance to ask a question, the line went dead. When Peter walked into the kitchen, Julie was still standing next to the phone. He had been putting Brittany to bed upstairs. "It's in her bones now," Julie said. "That's what happened with Mom. It got into her bones."

Peter walked over and hugged her. But his embrace felt oddly tentative. Julie was not sure whether Peter was offering solace or seeking it.

Jennifer's cancer stabilized for a few months in the spring, but one evening in May, Aunt Grace called with more bad news; she said that the doctors were concerned about a metastasis to the brain now. Jennifer was having an MRI the next day.

Julie felt a sharp pain in her stomach.

Was that the baby kicking? Or her body reacting to Grace's news?

"I'm glad you'll be there when Jennifer gets the results back," Grace said. She knew that Julie was due to visit Phoenix in a few days. "Someone from the family should be there."

Julie wanted to get off the phone. Here she was, thirty-four and pregnant—no Mackey woman had survived that set of circumstances for two generations now.

A few days later, Jennifer's husband, Rick, met Julie at Phoenix International Airport. In the parking lot, Rick stopped in front of a small black mini-bus and took out his keys. Julie was surprised. Jennifer had made the van sound huge, almost like a Mack truck, but the little mini-bus Rick was standing in front of was hardly bigger than a car. Julie, though well into her fifth month, was able to climb into the cab easily.

"You know what would take care of everything?" Julie said the next morning; they were sitting in Jennifer's kitchen waiting for the radiologist to call with the scan results. "A cheesecake."

Jennifer smiled. "A cheesecake, yes, a strawberry cheesecake."

In Huntingdon Valley the refrigerator had been the one dependable source of consolation for the sisters.

"No, no," Julie said. "Not strawberry. Lemon. A lemon cheesecake."

Jennifer started to say something, when the phone rang.

She picked it up: "Yes, it is" . . . pause . . . "All right, I'll wait." The nurse, Julie thought, must be getting the radiologist on the line. Jennifer looked over at her; they exchanged glances. "Hello," Jennifer said. The radiologist must be speaking now. ". . . Yes, Doctor . . . yes . . . I see . . . yes . . . I understand." It was bad news. Jennifer's voice sounded clogged, choked; she was struggling to maintain her self-control. ". . . Uh-huh . . . all right . . . no, no, I understand, Doctor . . . uh-huh . . . yes, Thursday . . . thank you, Doctor."

Jennifer hung up and turned to Julie.

"They found four spots in my brain."

The rest of that day had an oddly anticlimactic feel, like a class that goes on after the final exam is over. Julie does not remember much about it, except for a brief conversation she and Jennifer had a few hours later in the living room.

Jennifer said what frightened her most about dying was that her children would never know her. Deidre was only four, Melody two. She had not had enough time to finish her work with them, to put her maternal imprint on them. Deidre might remember her in a shadowy way, the way Julie remembered their mother. But Melody would never know her, would never feel any lasting emotional connection to her. She, Jennifer, would always be a face in a photograph to her younger child.

Going to bed that night, Julie thought about her own mother. Was that why Kay had wept so inconsolably in the waiting room that morning? Julie imagined that this knowledge, this awareness that the children you carried inside you, nurtured, and loved would not remember you, must be a death within death.

Julie's concern about Jennifer mounted through the summer, but after the uneventful birth of Mark Paul Conte one hot morning in early July 1994, she stopped worrying about herself. She was now past the danger period; Jennifer and Kay had both developed symptoms—notably breast pain—during pregnancy; Julie had had none. A cancer could always appear later, of course, but the doctors considered the possibility so remote, they did not recommend any special postpartum screening or monitoring procedures.

Between work, which she returned to in late August, and taking care of Mark and Brittany, September was a blur to Julie. But at the end of the month, Aunt Grace called to offer a respite: a weekend-long, all-sisters slumber party in Phoenix. Grace said everything was already taken care of. All Julie had to do was show up at the Phoenix Intercontinental Hotel at the start of the Columbus Day weekend.

Julie knew that the slumber party was a fiction. In June, Jennifer's oncologist, Paul Orenstein, had told Rick that Jennifer had only four or five months left. If Dr. Orenstein was right, the Columbus Day weekend would mark the start of her last month of life. The party was just an excuse Aunt Grace had invented to give the other sisters an opportunity to say good-bye to her. But everyone, including Julie, was happy to go along with the fiction. It was easier to think about than the truth.

Jennifer met the sisters in a wheelchair.

In July, she had made a public announcement about the wheelchair, but it was still a shock, walking into the lobby of the Phoenix Intercontinental and seeing her sitting in the chair. Watching Jennifer die was like watching someone sink helplessly into quicksand. The sand was up to her chin now. Soon, it would swallow her entirely.

"Remember what we promised each other," Julie told Lisa when they went upstairs to change. "No tears. We're going to be happy for Jennifer."

Generous portions of champagne along with the familiar rhythms of sisterhood helped make the promise easier to keep. Two hours later, a naked, squealing Julie was sitting in a bathtub with three other naked, squealing adult women. No one could remember the date of the Mackey sisters' last collective bath, but Jennifer said 1966 was probably a pretty good guess. Three days of massages, facials, hairdressers, shopping, and eating followed.

On the last night of the party, Jennifer made a reference to Dr. Orenstein's prognosis. "I know what he told Rick," she said as she and Julie were sitting on the hotel balcony watching the day fade away into the big desert sky. "But Orenstein's wrong. I'm going to have Deidre and Melody for one more Christmas. I'm going to see their faces on one more Christmas. God won't deprive me of that, Julie, I know he won't."

At the end of November, it appeared as if Dr. Orenstein had been right. On the twenty-seventh, Jennifer was rushed to the hospital. The news that reached Pennsylvania that night was grave in the extreme: Jennifer was in a coma, her survival doubtful.

But two days later, against all expectations, she rallied. She would live a little longer, though no one, including Dr. Orenstein, knew how much longer.

"Jennifer always was stubborn," Aunt Grace said that evening when she called Julie from Phoenix. Julie put the phone in the crook of her neck and squeezed the receiver against her shoulder. Then she lifted baby Mark out of the crib.

"Jennifer is stubborn," Julie agreed.

Jennifer came home from the hospital on December 10. Twelve days later, Emily flew to Phoenix.

Emily went to help Rick and Deidre and Melody through the holidays, but she also went to Arizona to bear witness; Jennifer was near the end of the end now, and Emily thought—hoped—that her presence, a sisterly presence, would help ease the last few days of Jennifer's life. But as the holidays approached, Jennifer's capacity to receive succor dwindled, diminished, then vanished. Long periods of sleep alternated with brief, confused moments of semi-delirium.

"I don't think she knows where she is anymore," Rick said on Christmas Eve.

But the next morning, Christmas morning, when Emily went in to check on Jennifer, Jennifer opened her eyes and said: "Are the kids up yet?"

"No," Emily whispered.

"What time is it?" Jennifer's voice was very weak.

"Seven. A little after."

"They'll be up soon. Take me into the living room. I want to be in the living room when they come downstairs."

Moving Jennifer was dangerous and painful. But this was the moment she had fought for.

"All right," Emily said. "Let me get Rick."

When Rick arrived, the two of them lifted Jennifer into a wheel-chair, then Emily wheeled her into the living room.

"There," Jennifer said. She pointed to a couch in front of the Christmas tree. "I'll be able to see everything from there."

Jennifer fell asleep on the couch. But as soon as the sound of running feet began to reverberate overhead, she opened her eyes. Emily was helping her sit up when Deidre and Melody burst into the living room.

The next hour was remarkably normal. Presents were ripped open, wrapping paper tossed in the air, new toys and clothing displayed and tried on. Jennifer had been granted her last wish.

At eleven, Emily wheeled her back to her room and gave her two pain pills. Almost immediately, Jennifer was asleep again.

Emily, Rick, and the children had dinner around six. Afterward, Deidre and Melody helped Emily stack the dirty dishes for the dishwasher, then went upstairs. Emily was still in the kitchen cleaning up when she heard a moan.

"Ooooohhhh."

At first Emily thought she had imagined the sound; it was very low. She took a dish off the counter and put it into the dishwasher.

"OOOOOHHHHHHH."

Emily slammed the dishwasher door shut and ran into Jennifer's room.

Rick was already there.

"Rick?"

"I don't know . . . I don't know . . ."

Jennifer was thrashing from side to side; her face and arms were dripping with perspiration. The veins in her neck, bulging and bright red, looked about to burst.

"Maybe she's in pain?" Rick said. "The night nurse will be here soon . . . at ten." Normally, Jennifer had around-the-clock nursing care. But the day nurse had taken Christmas Day off.

"OOOOHHHHHHHHHHHHHH."

Deidre and Melody! Emily thought. They must hear the moaning. What if this was their last memory of their mother? This awful moan.

Emily grabbed Rick's arm. "We have to get the kids out of here."

Rick wrote down a telephone number and gave it to Emily. "The Devereuxs," he said, "friends . . . call them . . . they should be home now."

Ten minutes later, the doorbell rang. Emily and Rick ran upstairs, woke the girls, and carried them down to the front hall. When Rick opened the door, the Devereuxs were standing on the porch, their car running in the driveway.

Just as Emily was helping the girls into their coats, there was another moan.

"OOOOOOOOOOOOOOOOOOOHHHHHHHHHHHHHHHHH-HHHHHHH."

The awful sound echoed up and down the quiet street. A dog began to bark.

Melody looked at Emily, but she didn't say anything. She didn't ask where the sound was coming from, or who was making it. "It's okay, baby," Emily whispered, "it's okay." Then she picked up Melody and dashed out the front door, Rick followed with Deidre.

When the night nurse arrived, she administered a dose of morphine. But the pain, stubborn and indomitable, did not abate. The moaning continued through the night and into the early morning. Around eight, there was a particularly awful moan; it rose higher and higher—then, just when it seemed about to burst through the roof, it stopped, and the house became perfectly still.

When Emily ran into Jennifer's room, Rick was standing by the bed, weeping and shaking.

"She's dead, Emily. My Jennifer is dead."

Everyone flew out for the funeral. Aunt Grace was there, of course; Julie, Emily, Lisa, Susan, and Bob Junior, and their respective spouses and boyfriends. After the service, Emily was standing on the church steps when she heard someone say, "I don't know how Rick did it." She turned around; Julie's husband, Peter, was standing beside her. "I could never go through what Rick went through," Peter said. "Never."

Julie and Peter were the last of the family to leave Phoenix. On New Year's Eve, Rick drove them out to the airport. The next day, they attended a small, cheerless New Year's Day gathering at Lisa's house in North Wales, Pennsylvania. When they arrived home in Newtown at nine, Julie went right to bed; she was exhausted.

The bedroom window was a sheet of white when she awoke the next morning. Last night, on the drive home, the radio had predicted heavy snow for today, six to eight inches. The alarm clock was still ringing. As Julie reached over to shut it off, she felt a sharp pain. She tried again. More pain. Worse this time. The alarm continued to ring.

Peter rolled over and opened his eyes. Julie was sitting up in the bed running her hands across her chest. She looked as if she had been struck.

"What's wrong?" Peter asked.

Julie burst into tears.

Peter bolted upright in the bed. "Julie, what's the matter?"

"I have a pain in my breast," Julie wailed.

CHAPTER THREE

JULIE'S HOUSE SITS ON THE RISE OF A HILL.

About a quarter of a mile below the house, her street, Jerusalem Road, flows into Old Darlington Road, an older, two-lane highway that winds lazily down the hill for another mile or so before passing a sprawling Dutch Colonial farmhouse. Stone-faced and white-framed, the farmhouse is a reminder of the Old Newtown, the Newtown of dairy farms and overhanging trees, of narrow, undulating roads with lovely old biblical names, and sleepy summer days, the Newtown that used to be before the subdivisions and the Burger Kings arrived.

At a little meadow just below the farmhouse, Old Darlington makes an abrupt right turn, then runs Kansas-flat for two hundred yards before intersecting with the Newtown Turnpike. At the northeast corner of the intersection, the Randall Peabody School sits unobtrusively behind a row of elms.

For Julie, the proximity to the school was one of the Jerusalem

Road house's major selling points. "I can drop the kids off on the way to work," she told Peter the day they looked at the house.

On this morning, the first workday of the new year, 1995, that conversation seemed a thousand years away.

"I'm sure it's nothing," Peter said. He was watching Julie put on her coat. The door behind her led to the driveway. "You probably just twisted something shutting off the alarm clock."

Julie said she was calling the doctor anyway, as soon as she got to St. Monica's Hospital, where she was a public affairs officer.

Driving down the hill, Julie began to threaten, wheedle, bargain with God, fate, Jennifer's ghost, herself—Julie was not sure whom she was addressing. She was only sure of one thing: breast cancer had made a big mistake if it had chosen Julie Conte as its next victim.

Others could unfurl the battle flags and beat the drums, but let the word go out: In the war against breast cancer, Julie Conte was opting out. She was burning her draft card and fleeing across the border to Canada.

As Julie was making a right at the Peabody School intersection, slush from a passing LandCruiser blinded her. She pulled over to the side of the road and opened the glove compartment. No rags—have to use one of Mark's Pampers to wipe off the windshield. Julie reached into the backseat and took a diaper out of the box.

No pain!

Maybe Peter was right, after all.

The only hypothesis Peter had been willing to entertain this morning was the funny-twist hypothesis, that and the psychosomatic hypothesis: Either Julie had turned awkwardly while shutting off the alarm clock or she had imagined the pain. "It would be perfectly normal," Peter said in advancing the second hypothesis. Pulling back into the snowy morning traffic, Julie felt a rush of panic. Oh my God, she thought, what am I gonna do if I have it?

.   .   .

"It's just a precaution," Julie's family doctor, Philip Lamangelli,* said that night. Even though he had failed to find anything, Dr. Lamangelli wanted Julie to see a breast surgeon. "With your history," he said, "I think we have to be supercareful." He recommended a Dr. Lawrence Winters* at Albert Einstein Medical Center in Philadelphia. Dr. Lamangelli said Julie should get a mammogram done before she saw the surgeon. The next morning, she called a radiology center in Lansdale and made an appointment.

Dr. Winters was a large, cheerful, white-haired man.

Julie removed her mammogram from a manila folder and passed it across the desk. Dr. Winters glanced at it briefly, then smiled at Julie. He said he understood that she had a family history of breast cancer.

"My mother and sister both died of the disease," Julie said. "My sister just died a few weeks ago."

It was January twentieth. Twenty-six days after Jennifer's death.

Dr. Winters picked up a folder and opened it. He read the first page of the file, then looked at Julie. "You had a pain in your chest on January second?"

"Yes, right here." Julie pointed to her breastbone. "I haven't felt it since."

The surgeon said it was highly unusual to have disease in the breastbone. He smiled again.

"I know I could have imagined the pain," Julie said.

"That would certainly be understandable, Julie."

Dr. Winters's hands moved across Julie's breasts expertly, quickly. Lots of approving head nods. Julie could feel her fear beginning to lift. The surgeon walked over to his desk and made a notation in Julie's file; then he picked up the mammogram again and looked at it. Julie was sure that Dr. Winters was about to cast his vote for the psychosomatic hypothesis.

But Dr. Winters surprised her; he chose a different hypothesis.

"Here, let me show you. You can see it."

Dr. Winters had beautiful fingers, long, supple, elegant. At the moment, one of those exquisite fingers was sliding across the mammogram; it stopped at a shadowy white object on the left side near the border. The object had a funny shape; it was sort of an irregular circle. Julie studied it carefully. It was small, which was good, but it was also light, which was not good. Healthy breast tissue photographs dark on a mammogram.

Dr. Winters said he wanted to palpate Julie's left breast again. The object was located on the left breast near the armpit.

This time the surgeon felt an irregularity. "Have you ever had a breast aspiration?" he asked.

Julie felt light-headed. Not enough oxygen. Something was wrong with her breathing.

Julie said no.

The surgeon smiled. "No big deal. I do aspirations all the time, Julie." Dr. Winters's deep, rich baritone was reassuring.

"I'll give you a little anesthetic. You won't feel a thing."

Dr. Winters was right. There was only a tingling sensation when the needle pierced the skin. Julie ignored it; she was studying the diplomas above Dr. Winters's desk. He had two from the University of Pennsylvania, one from the college and one from the medical school. Dr. Winters also had a certificate from the American College of Surgeons. The certificate said that Dr. Winters was a diplomate of the college.

Julie examined the embossed gold leafing on the certificate, then looked down at her breast. The needle was almost all the way inside now; only about a half inch of very thin steel protruded above the skin. A mass of fluid suddenly spurted to the top of the cylinder. The fluid was translucent, except for a few little red spots near the top of the cylinder. The spots looked like little crimson ink stains.

Dr. Winters looked up. "You had me worried for a minute, Julie. I wasn't sure this thing was going to give up any fluid." Cysts were wet, the surgeon explained, solid tumors usually dry.

"Now you tell me you were worried."

Dr. Winters smiled. "I'm the one who's supposed to do the worrying around here, Julie. That's why they pay me the big bucks."

"Everything's all right, then?" Julie asked.

A definitive diagnosis would require laboratory analysis, Dr. Winters said. But it was definitely a good sign, the fluid. There was also a bad sign, but Dr. Winters did not mention that until Julie called his office a week later.

Julie knew something was wrong right away.

The nurse would not release her lab results; she said Dr. Winters wanted to speak to Julie personally. He was with a patient now. "Where can we reach you, Mrs. Conte?" Julie gave the nurse her work number.

Why did Dr. Winters want to talk her personally? Julie wondered.

Maybe he wanted to apologize? Maybe someone in the surgeon's office had misplaced Julie's breast fluid and now a profoundly embarrassed Dr. Winters wanted to apologize for the error. Julie put down the phone. A cyst also was a possibility. A definite possibility. A cyst would produce a positive laboratory result, wouldn't it? Of course it would.

At a quarter of two, the phone on Julie's desk rang. Julie whispered a little prayer and picked it up.

"Julie. How are you?"

Dr. Winters.

"We have the test results back."

The little blood vessels behind Julie's ears began to dilate wildly. How did her heart get into her brain?

"Remember when I said I was glad I got fluid out?"

"Yes," Julie said.

"I was glad," Dr. Winters said. "But when I saw blood in the fluid, I was concerned."

The little red ink stains. Damn, now Julie's heart was trying to burst through her skull. She put her hand on top of her head to hold it in.

"There were some malignant cells in the fluid, Julie."

"How bad is it?" Was that her voice? Impossible, Julie thought. No one could speak at a moment like this. *Malignant cells*—Jesus!

"Is it really bad, Dr. Winters?" Her voice again. Amazing.

"I don't know anything yet, Julie. I can't answer any questions until we do more tests."

Julie tried again. "How frightened should I be?"

"I'm sorry, Julie, I need more information."

Either the surgeon could not hear Julie crying, or he decided to ignore it. He told her to call Dr. Lamangelli at five. "I'm going to talk to him now. He'll tell you what tests I want you to have. Speak to you soon."

When she hung up, Julie looked through the glass partition in her office. No one in the outer office was staring, no one was whispering. No one must have seen her crying. Julie removed a Kleenex from her purse, wiped her eyes very quickly, then picked up the phone and called Peter.

The stolid, sensible Peter answered. The Peter Aunt Grace called the strong, silent type, the Peter Julie herself described as "a man's man," the Peter who would never let you down, the Peter who was a rock, the Peter all Julie's single friends wanted to marry.

"You have to remain calm," this Peter said. "You're not Jennifer. Everything will be all right." Julie was very fond of this sensible Peter. But she did not want to talk to him today. Today, Julie wanted to talk to the other Peter, the frightened, emotional Peter. The Peter of the tentative hug in the kitchen and the whispered question in the bedroom, the Peter who would break down and cry when Julie told him she had breast cancer. But that Peter was not in the office today.

Julie dialed another number. A man in the outer office picked up the phone on his desk. Julie watched him through the glass.

"Mike, do you have a minute?" Mike Kimecko was Julie's best friend at work.

Mike smiled at Julie from his desk.

"What's up?" Mike sounded as if he were in Peru, but his face was only fifty feet away on the other side of the glass.

Julie tried to speak, but could not. She began to cry into the phone.

"It was positive," Julie said, when Mike walked into her office.

When Mike and Julie hugged, Betty Frederick, the head of the public affairs department, got up and walked into Julie's office. "What's the matter?" she asked.

When Betty and Julie hugged, Colleen McGuillicudy, another PA officer, got up and went into Julie's office. Colleen also hugged Julie when she heard the news. In the larger office outside, work had come to a stop. Julie's breast cancer was becoming public news.

Julie felt odd as the staff, most of them new, began to drift into her office to offer condolences. This was supposed to be a profoundly intimate moment, a profoundly personal moment, and here were people Julie barely knew telling her how sorry they were, how terrible it was, how much they cared for her.

Julie felt like Rocky leaving the office. People jostled with one another to touch her, to feel her hand, to pat her on the back, to wish her well. "I'll pray for you, Julie," complete strangers shouted. "I'll say a Rosary for you, I'll offer up a novena, have a Mass said."

At the day care center, the staff sensed that something was wrong, since Julie arrived two hours early. But nobody pried or asked difficult questions. One of the day care workers, a heavyset, grandmotherly woman named Edna, wrestled Brittany into her coat, then carried Mark out to the car for Julie.

At the Jerusalem Road turnoff, a gust of wind shook the car. The windows rattled, then everything turned white. Suddenly, it began to snow furiously.

Julie pulled over to the side of the road and looked into the back-seat again.

Brittany was awake.

"You okay, baby?"

Brittany looked at the rattling, clattering windows and started to cry. A startled Mark opened his eyes and let out a wail. Then Julie began to cry again.

She removed a handkerchief from her purse and reached over the front seat. No pain again!

The pain had turned out to be an illusion after all. Winters had said so this afternoon. "No, Julie," he had said. "You imagined the pain in your cleavage. The tumor is located near the armpit on the other side of your breast." But Winters could believe what he wanted. Julie was sure about the pain. Absolutely sure. On January second, her sister Jennifer had sent a warning down from heaven. The pain had been a heavenly communication designed to get Julie to Lamangelli and Winters before her cancer had a chance to spread.

Now Julie was sure Jennifer was putting in a good word for her.

"Julie's so young, God . . . and her children . . . they're babies. They need Julie now. You can't take their mother away. Besides, God, twice in one family is enough."

Julie wiped Brittany's eyes, then Mark's, then her own.

At dinner, Peter was as controlled as the Peter on the phone.

"We don't want to get ahead of the curve," he said.

Julie could not understand it. Peter looked normal. Not one sign of fear in his face. Not one.

"All we know now is that there are some malignant cells in your breast fluid, Julie. We don't know if you have a growth . . . we don't even know if you have cancer. Winters said malignant cells, didn't he? He didn't say cancer."

"No," Julie agreed. "He didn't say cancer."

"All right, then, let's not get ahead of the curve."

Julie nodded. She was not listening. She was thinking about the curve, trying to imagine what it looked like. Whatever it looked like, Julie was sure that she was always going to be ahead of it. Even if they put it on roller skates, even if it sprouted wings, even if they attached rocket engines to the curve, it would never catch up to Julie Conte. Never.

"Snow," Brittany said. She was sitting between her parents in a high chair. Her mouth was covered with tapioca pudding.

Peter smiled. "That's right, honey. Snow."

Brittany pointed her spoon at the window. "Snow," she said again.

Peter smiled. "Big snow."

Julie looked out the window. Too dark to see now . . . nearly seven. But Brittany was right. According to the weatherman, snow through Sunday morning. Near-blizzard conditions from Maine to Georgia.

Dr. Lamangelli was gone when Julie called at five; a voice on the answering machine said the office had closed early because of the weather and would not reopen until Monday morning. Monday morning was fifty hours away. Fifty hours snowbound with two small children, a strange shadowy object in her breast, and no information. Julie was convinced that she could not survive fifty hours under those conditions. No one could. At hour twenty or thirty Julie was going to explode or go crazy or dissolve into molten ash or kill someone.

Peter was talking about second opinions now, about how important they are. "We have to think this through," Peter said. "We have to plan, Julie. We need a plan."

"What if I need a mastectomy?" Julie asked. "How would you feel about that, about having a wife with one breast?"

The question caught Peter off guard.

He looked over at Brittany. She was struggling with her spoon. Peter reached over and helped her, then turned back to Julie. "A mastectomy would not change anything."

"What about sex?" Julie asked. "How would you feel making love to a woman with one breast?"

Peter put his hand on Julie's. "Look, we'll get through this somehow. I know we will. . . . I know you will."

"Jennifer didn't."

"Stop that, Julie. You're not Jennifer. You're you."

"Lucky me."

Saturday morning.

Julie opened her eyes and looked out the window. Still snowing. Julie rolled over. Peter was asleep. He must have slept funny; his cowlick was all spiky. He looked like Spanky in the old *Our Gang* comedies. Julie reached over and smoothed down his hair, then got up, put on her housecoat, and went downstairs.

The coffee filters were in the kitchen cabinet over the sink. Julie took the box down and opened it. Where had she read about video messages? One of the women's magazines? Julie could not remember. She opened the box and took out a cone-shaped filter. Leave your child with a living memory, that was the idea. A video message would show what Mommy or Daddy actually looked and sounded like. Of course, you would need a video camera. But what would she say in her video message? Mark was only six months old. What do you say to a baby? "I love you," of course, but what else?

Julie picked up the coffee canister.

"I'm sorry I died on you, Mark. But please, honey, don't be mad at me. I didn't mean to die. Honest. It wasn't my fault. I didn't desert you. Things happen. You'll understand when you get older."

Julie opened a kitchen drawer. Big spoon or little spoon? Peter liked strong coffee; she did not. Julie picked a little spoon.

Brittany's message would be harder. Brittany would be angry at her. Furious. How could Brittany not be furious? How could any daughter not be furious? Julie put the filter holder on top of the coffeepot. "I'm sorry, Brittany. You know I didn't want to make you go through this. You know that, baby, don't you? Forgive your mother. I love you. I love you, baby. Love your mother back. Please." Julie picked up the spoon and began to scoop coffee into the filter.

"Maybe you won't get it, Brittany. Maybe you won't get breast cancer. Maybe by the time you see this video there will be a cure already. Forgive your mother, baby. Say you forgive her. Say you love her. I love you."

CHAPTER FOUR

DEMOGRAPHERS ESTIMATE THAT BETWEEN 69 AND 110 BILLION PEO-
ple have walked the earth. The discrepancy between the high and low
estimates reflects a disagreement about when to start the human cen-
sus. Biblical literalists begin 6,000 years ago, when (according to Old
Testament calculations) Adam and Eve entered the Garden of Eden.
Academic demographers start a million years ago, or roughly midway
between the emergence of genus *Homo sapiens*, an erect, tool-bearing
people, and ancient *Homo erectus*, our next-to-last direct ancestor.

For most of time, anonymity has been a constant of the human condition. Most of our ancestors lived and died as anonymously as a blade
of grass lives and dies. Alex Shulmatoff, author of *A Mountain of
Names*, estimates that only a handful, maybe only 6 to 7 billion, of the
69 to 110 billion people who have ever lived, have left behind any
record of their existence. Most often the record consists of a name
scrawled hurriedly on some daily piece of business—a parish marriage
record, or a contract with a neighboring farmer for a cow or a bushel of
wheat.

The Utah Genealogical Society, an arm of the Church of Jesus Christ of Latter-day Saints, is the largest collector of human names in the world. Latter-day Saints, or Mormons, do not believe that people die—at least, not in a spiritual sense. All the people who have ever lived are, in the Mormon view, still alive; they reside, all 69 to 110 billion of them, in a vast spirit world where they wait for someone to call their names. Mormons believe that special covenants or pacts can be made with a relative in the spirit world if the relative's name is known to you.

To help church members locate kin in the spirit world, the Utah Genealogical Society has collected nearly 2 billion names at its Granite Mountain Vault in Salt Lake City. The names, which come from all places and all times and all races of the human family, represent a kind of great chain of being. The chain stretches backward and forward in time until it connects nearly every human being to nearly every other human being. In 1994, the chain intersected with Julie's name and with Jennifer's and with the names of their sisters, and with the name of every other woman who has ever had a family history of breast cancer, and possibly with the name of every woman who has had or will ever have the disease. The intersection occurred when a group of Granite Mountain names led researchers out on to the long arm of chromosome 17, and to a genetic marker known as 17q21-22, which lives in the same genetic neighborhood as BRCA 1, the familial breast cancer gene.

Hippocrates, who seemed to notice everything, noticed that certain cancers, including breast cancer, run in families. Pierre Paul Broca, the nineteenth-century French surgeon, noticed so many things about the human neurological system that he has an area of the brain named after him, Broca's area, and a medical condition, Broca's aphasia, which is a form of speech dysfunction caused by lesions in Broca's area.

Broca's work in the field of cancer is less well known, but almost as remarkable. In the 1840s, at the age of twenty-five, he became the first scientist to argue that cancer cells can metastasize through the venous (blood) system; a quarter of a century later, Broca also became the first physician to describe a case of familial breast cancer. The family was his in-laws, the Lugols; in *Traités des Tumeurs*, Broca reported that, between 1788 and 1858, the Lugol family experienced a total of thirty-eight cancer deaths. The Lugol women accounted for twenty-four and most of them died of breast cancer, though gastrointestinal malignancies were also common.

Broca suspected that a heredity factor was involved in this terrible history. But in 1865, when *Traités des Tumeurs* was published, the mechanisms of heredity were as unknown as the dark side of the moon.

Around the same time *Traités* was published, an Austrian monk, Gregor Mendel, was creating the foundations of modern genetic theory in a monastery garden with his sweet pea experiments. But oddly, until the 1970s, Mendelian genetic theory was only occasionally applied to the study of familial breast cancer. In 1946, a Dutch researcher named David Jacobsen confirmed Broca's observation about the high incidence of other cancers in some breast cancer families. Jacobsen's report was called "Heredity and Breast Cancer."

In the late 1960s, interest in familial breast cancer began to quicken. In 1970, David Anderson, an oncologist at M. D. Anderson Hospital in Houston, asked a question so simple that it was a wonder no one had thought to ask it before: How does a family history of breast cancer affect a woman's personal risk? After examining the records of 500 patients, Anderson concluded the risk was selective. The personal risk rate barely moves when a second-degree relative (e.g., a cousin) develops the disease, but rises significantly when two first-degree relatives, say, a mother and a sister, are stricken.

Around the same time, Henry Lynch, a Creighton University investigator, asked another simple question: How many forms of familial breast cancer are there? This question had been asked before, but Lynch's answer was the most sophisticated to date. He identified three hereditary forms of the disease. Some breast cancer families, like the Lugols, also have a high incidence of gastrointestinal tumors; some, a high incidence of ovarian cancers; and some, like Julie's family, the Mackeys, have breast cancer alone.

In 1971, an investigator named Alfred Knudson asked the most basic question of all: How does a hereditary predisposition lead to cancer? Knudson, then a pediatrician and geneticist at M. D. Anderson in Houston, asked the question about retinoblastoma (RB), another hereditary malignancy. But medicine's understanding of all familial cancers would be changed by Knudson's discoveries about hereditary RB.

Retinoblastoma, which can produce bulging tumors in the retina of the eye, is, like other pediatric cancers, blessedly rare. The incidence is one in every 20,000 births and the usual age of onset is two. On occasion, however, a baby will be born with a tumor in the eye because retinoblastoma, like breast and fifty other types of cancer, comes in a hereditary, as well as a nonhereditary form.

RB's early onset puzzled Knudson. How could a newborn have enough time to develop an eye tumor? According to the multi-hit theory, the prevailing theory of cancer growth, three to seven individual mutations ("hits") are needed to make a cell cancerous. Since fifty or sixty years is enough time for a combination of environmental carcinogens and normally occurring biological mistakes to deliver five or six hits to a cell, the multi-hit theory made sense as an explanation for adult cancer. But Knudson did not think that it was of much sense for a pediatric cancer like RB, which could be present at birth.

Could fewer hits, perhaps many fewer hits, also produce a malignancy?

Knudson thought so. Beginning in 1971 with a paper called "Mutation and Cancer: Statistical Study of Retinoblastoma," he began to develop a two-hit theory of cancer to explain RB. Besides fewer steps, Knudson's theory also contained one other novel element. Retinoblastoma, the researcher said, was triggered not by an oncogene, which produces wild cell proliferation, but by a different—and in the early 1970s, still unidentified—genetic mechanism.

Even if all environmental carcinogens disappeared tomorrow, cancer would continue (though at perhaps one-fifth its present rate), because genes would continue to mutate spontaneously, i.e., naturally. The normal mutation rate for each gene is one mistake per every million cell divisions; in other words, once in every million divisions the body makes an error and produces a mutant copy of a gene. Knudson believed that hereditary RB originated in such a mutation; it occurred in a gene now known as RB.

Today, RB would be called a tumor suppressor gene, and it acts the way p53 seems to act during the adolescent growth spurt, as a kind of control mechanism or brake on cellular growth. Just as osteoblast cells proliferate rapidly during the growth spurt, during the retina's creation, retinoblasts proliferate rapidly. RB keeps the growth process orderly and under control. Which is to say, it keeps rapid cellular proliferation from veering out of control and becoming disorderly and cancerlike. However, tumor suppressor genes, like all other genes, are subject to hits, or mutations, during cell division. But since genes come in pairs— we get one copy from each parent—a single hit is rarely dangerous, because a backup copy of the regulator gene immediately steps in to take over the braking function.

Dr. Knudson's work continues to be influential because he was the first investigator to explain how a hereditary hit produces a familial predisposition to cancer. In the case of the retinoblastoma gene, Dr. Knudson said, the child with a hereditary predisposition receives a good copy of the RB regulator gene from one parent and a bad, already mutated copy from the other parent. The defective RB gene, which may have first mutated hundreds of years ago in an ancestor, constitutes the first hit in the two-hit model of familial cancer. But the first hit, the hereditary hit, only creates a predisposition; one bad RB gene, one bad any regulator gene, does not create a cancer. A second hit has to occur; the good regulator gene has to be knocked out, too.

According to Dr. Knudson, the reason the second, "good" RB gene often takes a hit during the construction of the fetal retina is rapid cell proliferation, which is to a gene what driving through a thunderstorm is to a motorist, a period of heightened vulnerability to accident. The millions of cell divisions required to build a retina increase the odds that the good RB gene will sustain a mutation or be destroyed. Knudson said familial retinoblastoma often appears very early, because 90 to 95 percent of children with an inherited mutation take a hit in utero or some time soon thereafter. Once that happens, once both RB regulators have been destroyed or knocked out, the journey to retinoblastoma is brief, because mutant cells are now free to grow in a wild, unregulated, cancerlike fashion.

"Mutation and Cancer," Knudson's first formulation of the two-hit model, was published in the February 8, 1971, issue of the *Proceedings of the National Academy of Sciences*. Initially, the paper did not attract much attention. But within a few years, Knudson's logic, which was spare and elegant, began to win adherents.

However, even Knudson's most enthusiastic supporters believed that the two-hit model was applicable to pediatric cancers only. Dozens, perhaps even hundreds, of genes played a role in the rise of such complex adult familial carcinomas as breast cancer. Everyone was sure of it. Or almost everyone.

A few weeks before the 1990 meeting of the American Society of Human Genetics was due to convene in Cincinnati, Berkeley geneticist Mary-Claire King called Louise Strong, a member of the ASHG board, and asked to be included among the meeting's speakers. King said she had an important finding to announce.

The request was unusual but the board decided to grant it anyway. In 1972, King had startled the scientific community with her discovery that man and chimp share more than 99 percent of their DNA. Maybe she had another startling announcement to make now? She did. A few weeks later, in a Cincinnati hotel auditorium overflowing with geneticists and journalists, King announced that she and her team had discovered the general location of a gene that conferred a heightened risk of breast cancer on a carrier. The gene was called BRCA, for breast cancer gene, and while its workings were still unclear, the King gene appeared to operate like the Knudson RB gene. Which is to say, it was a mutant variety of a regulator gene, passed on from family member to family member, and was singlehandedly capable of producing a predisposition to cancer. King said that while she and her team had tracked the gene to the long arm of chromosome 17, they had not yet been able to identify its exact location on the arm.

King's last announcement set off one of the most exciting and contentious races in modern science.

Breast cancer, the second leading cause of cancer death among American women, strikes 184,000 women every year and kills 46,000 of them. Of the cancers, only those of the lung kill more women, 53,000 annually. It is estimated that 1.6 to 2.6 million (the higher figure includes undiagnosed cases) women currently live with breast cancer. And like Julie, 5 to 10 percent are thought to have a familial form of the disease.

Fifty-five is the average age of first diagnosis and 75 percent of breast cancer deaths occur among women in the fifty-five-and-up age group. But the death rate among older women is higher, because older women get breast cancer more often, not because they get a more virulent form of the disease. Just the opposite, in fact: In mature women, indolent, or slowly growing, cancers are more common. The most lethal cancers usually appear in premenopausal women, women in their twenties, thirties, and early forties.

Peter A. Spratt, a University of Louisville surgeon, has found astounding variation in the aggressiveness of breast cancer. According to Spratt, some breast tumors can double in size in as little as ten days, while others take nearly twenty years to increase twofold in mass (260 days is the average doubling time for a breast tumor). Studies such as Spratt's are at the foundation of a new view of the disease. Proponents believe that, in terms of course and lethality, breast cancer really should be considered three different diseases. Dr. Peter Wasson of Dartmouth Medical School defines the three breast cancers this way.

He calls the first type, the type younger women usually get, "mean." Wasson says: "This breast cancer spreads so quickly, current technology cannot detect it or treat it. Something is wrong at the cellular level and the cells spread rapidly throughout the body." According to Wasson, "The second type of breast cancer grows more slowly but at a fast enough rate to cause trouble . . . within a relatively short time—five to ten years." The third type is the most benign type. "It may take even longer to spread if it spreads at all," says Wesson.

Whatever form it takes, all breast cancer is genetically driven. And until King's announcement in Cincinnati, the two genes most frequently implicated in the disease were Her/2 neu and p53.

Her/2 neu is involved in the production of growth-factor receptors. The receptors, which sit on the cell surface like tiny satellite dishes, receive growth messages from the cellular internet. In 1986 Dr. Dennis Slamon of UCLA found that about 25 to 30 percent of breast cancers possess a mutant variety of Her/2 neu. Slamon also found that cancer cells with the Her/2 neu mutation frequently have extra copies of the healthy Her/2 neu gene, sometimes as many as twenty or thirty extra copies. Many investigators believe that these healthy genes may account for the often aggressive character of Her/2 neu–linked breast cancer.

The reason: The more Her/2 neu genes, the more growth-receptor sites a cell can make, and the more sites it makes, the more growth hormone it can receive, which enhances the cell's ability to multiply and divide.*

Pre-BRCA, the other gene most frequently implicated in breast cancer was p53. *Science* magazine's Molecule of the Year in 1993 and a *Newsweek* cover subject in 1996, p53 is the movie-star gene. What Elizabeth Taylor and Rosanne are to the tabloids, p53 is to the scien-

*In June 1998, Dr. Slamon reported that a new gene therapy developed to treat woman with Her/2 neu breast cancer had performed promisingly in clinical trials.

tific media. Over 5,000 papers have been devoted to the gene in the past decade. The astonishing notoriety of p53 comes in part from its astonishing ubiquity. Like Waldo, it seems to turn up everywhere. To date, it has been implicated in fifty-two different kinds of cancers, including breast, liver, and lung cancer, melanoma, lymphoma, and osteosarcoma.

Unlike Her/2 neu, an oncogene, p53 is a tumor suppressor gene, and in an unmutated state, it appears to regulate orderly, healthy cellular growth in two ways: p53 has a Dr. Kevorkian function; it assists in the suicide of potentially dangerous mutant cells and it also seems to help salvage damaged cells. When a mutation occurs, p53—with the help of several other genes—can order an injured cell to stop dividing until it has been repaired.

Gene p53 is implicated in 30 to 40 percent of breast cancers, but how it helps to foster the disease is not well understood. Sometimes it may be a case of wrong place, wrong time. The transcription of DNA to RNA is a key early step in cell division. Normally, p53 regulates the transcription process from within the cell nucleus. But in some breast cancer cells, the gene is unable to get to the nucleus. This means the unsupervised DNA can make any kind of crazy RNA it wants, and the RNA, which contains instructions for the manufacture of the new cell, can then make any kind of crazy cell it wants.

Despite the discovery of p53 and Her/2 neu, through the 1980s most scientists continued to believe that breast cancer, in its hereditary as well as its nonhereditary form, was too complex to be caused by any single gene.

Mary-Claire King still remembers the names of all the multigene proponents. During a recent interview with Kevin Davies, editor of *Nature Genetics*, King reeled them off. Anthony Murphy of Johns Hopkins, Raymond White of the University of Utah, and Eric Lander of MIT's Whitehead Institute. King's list read like a who's who of modern genetics. King told Davies that she remembered something else about the multigene proponents. They were all "boys."

Besides King, the only other major opponent of the multigene theory was Dr. Knudson, who in 1976 became a senior scientist at the Fox Chase Cancer Center in Philadelphia, an institution that Julie would become familiar with.

In a 1985 paper called "Hereditary Cancer: Oncogenes and Anti-Oncogenes," published in *Cancer Research*, Dr. Knudson hypothesized about the characteristics of the putative "breast cancer gene." He said it was not unreasonable to suppose that such a gene might mimic the action of the RB gene. That is, it might originate in an ancestral mutation, be transmitted from generation to generation within a family, and create a predisposition to breast cancer but not actually cause the disease.

Five years later, King would prove Knudson correct. And nine years later, after a bruising competition, a geneticist named Mark Skolnick (and several dozen names from the Granite Mountain Vault), would identify the breast cancer gene.

There are 100,000 genes in the human genome. This is the sum total of who we are. One hundred thousand genes plus environment equals us, humankind. The way geneticists such as King navigate through the genome is via chemical sequences known as markers. Markers make good navigational guides because they occur at predictable points along each of the forty-six chromosomes in the same way that directional signs occur at predictable points along a highway (for instance, before exits). Markers, which are heritable, also have another characteristic, one which makes them good gene-hunting tools as well as good directional guides. They vary from person to person and this variability makes it possible to do genetic comparisons.

For example, if the family members with an inherited disease share a marker at a particular site on a chromosome that is different in size and shape from the marker shared by healthy family members at the site, then two conclusions can reasonably be made: (a) a gene is probably involved in the family disease, and (b) the gene is probably located in the same general area of the chromosome as the marker.

In order to do such comparisons, however, you have to know where the markers are located.

Today, approximately 10,000 sites have been identified on the forty-six human chromosomes. But in 1987, when King began looking for the breast cancer gene, fewer than 100 sites had been identified. In effect, for the better part of next three years, she was wandering around a vast inner space with a map that had less than 100 place names on it. In human terms this is like trying to circumnavigate the globe on a vast ocean-spanning superhighway where the thousands of exits between Berlin and New Delhi or Anchorage and Lima are unmarked.

King could easily have spent several lifetimes circling round and round inside the human genome. But in the summer of 1990, quite by chance, she arrived at marker D17S74 on the long arm of chromosome 17. Her first step was to summon up the dead. You can use the DNA of living family members to reconstruct the chromosomal markers of ancestors, sometimes even very distant ancestors. King did this first. After she knew what kinds of markers her subjects' great-great-grandmothers and -aunts had at site D17S74, she compared them to the markers of her subjects. King got a partial match. Some of her living breast cancer patients had the same kind of marker at site D17S74 as family members who had died of the disease fifty or seventy years ago. Some, but not all.

One of King's assistants, a young geneticist named Beth Newman, helped to solve the puzzle. Since familial breast cancer usually strikes early, Newman suggested analyzing the family data by age. Immediately, everything fell into place. In the seven cases where a breast cancer had appeared early, before age forty-five, the data indicated the presence of a disease gene in the same general area as the D17S74 marker. "In this younger group," says King, "we saw physical evidence of . . . a specific ancient chromosome . . . that was descended from a common ancestor who lived anywhere from 150 to 2,000 years ago."

King's discovery had now narrowed the search for BRCA to a chromosomal area roughly equivalent to the area of Los Angeles County. To find the gene itself, she and everyone else who wanted to find it would have to search all of L.A. County for a single house, with no information about the house except that it had a red front door. However, everyone in the genetics community knew that the first person to knock at the red front door would be richly rewarded. There would be honor, acclaim, and of course, generous funding for future research projects. BRCA was an immensely important disease gene. Some researchers even believed it might play an important role in "normal" breast cancers, i.e., the nonfamilial kind.

Within three months of King's Cincinnati announcement, congestion was already becoming a problem on the long arm of chromosome 17. There were, besides King, a half dozen research teams—some from Europe, some from the United States—out on the arm, flashlights in hand. Before the race was over, a half dozen more teams would join the hunt, among them a Utah epidemiologist-turned-geneticist named Mark Skolnick.

In genetics, says Mary-Claire King, "The greatest advantage [goes to the person who has] accurate information on a large number of families." King's statement attests to the sheer power of numbers in genetic research. Simply put, the more families you have, the more chromosomal marker comparisons you can do. And the more comparisons you can do, the greater your chances of finding something important. Skolnick, who had access to the Mormons' Granite Mountain Vault, entered the race with more families than anyone else. In the late 1970s, he cross-referenced the names of 170,000 families in the vault with the names in the Utah cancer registry, creating one of the largest cancer databases in the world.

Skolnick also had another important advantage—money. In 1991, Skolnick left the University of Utah to cofound a company called Myriad Genetics, which raised $10 million to fund a private pursuit of BRCA 1.

The two advantages propelled Skolnick into a quick and, as it turned out, decisive lead. In early August 1994, a senior member of the Skolnick team, Donna Shattuck-Eiden, discovered a like mutation in several Myriad families on a gene at a site on chromosome 17q21-22. BRCA had been found.

A few days after Myriad announced victory, Natalie Angier of *The New York Times* wrote that scientists had captured "a genetic trophy so ferociously coveted and loudly heralded that it had taken on a near mythic aura."

In most of the hundreds of new stories written about the race's end, however, one important detail was omitted. The real work on BRCA was just beginning. Today, researchers all over the world are struggling to answer four basic questions.

The first is about the gene's relationship to ethnicity.

Ashkenazi Jewish women carry four specific BRCA mutations; the most common is 185delAG, which creates a predisposition to breast cancer *and* ovarian cancer. More recently, another specific BRCA mutation has been found in Icelandic women.

Dr. Knudson thinks similar discoveries may lie ahead. "Everyone with the 185 mutation," he notes, "has a common ancestor, who lived 500 to 1,000 years ago. I think one day we may also discover a distinctive German and Czech and Irish mutation and find that the women who share it also share a common ancestor."

Also yet to be answered is the question of how BRCA works.

Animal studies show that BRCA, like other tumor suppressor genes, is particularly active during periods of high breast cell division and growth, like pregnancy and adolescence. But how BRCA regulates cell growth, which is to say, how it suppresses mutant cells, is unclear. Some investigators believe it can order a hit cell to stop dividing until the hit damage has been repaired, while others believe the gene controls the operation of several subsidiary regulatory genes.

Yet to be clarified, as well, is the degree of risk BRCA confers on a woman.

The most often quoted risk figure is 85 percent over a lifetime, but recent research suggests that some carriers may have a lower risk. There are dozens of different kinds of BRCA mutations, and a woman's individual risk may be determined by the type of mutation she has.

The biggest unanswered question of all involves BRCA's role in "normal" breast cancer, and so far the evidence on this point is contradictory.

In 1995, a second breast cancer gene, BRCA 2, was identified. But many investigators, including Mary-Claire King, worry that there may be a BRCA 3 and even a BRCA 4.

"We're still not entirely sure what's going on," says King.

CHAPTER FIVE

Dr. Winters removed the mammogram from a manila folder and put it on his desk. Through the window, Julie could see a snow-plow clearing a space in front of the Einstein Medical Center. It was the Wednesday after the snowstorm and the Contes had driven into Philadelphia for a consultation. From her first visit, Julie vaguely remembered the looming gray presence of Einstein across the street, but not the high, paned windows or the stained parquet floors or the oriental rug under her chair. The surgeon's office looked like a Polo ad.

Dr. Winters slid the mammogram across the desk toward Peter. "Breast cancer usually doesn't look like this, Mr. Conte." He pointed to something on the left side of the photograph. "This is a very unusual configuration."

Julie looked out the window again. There were a group of women huddled near the entrance to Einstein, smoking. She watched them for a moment, then turned around. Peter was still hunched over the mammogram. But Dr. Winters was staring at her.

"I'm still not entirely convinced you have cancer, Julie. It's rare, but occasionally we do get a false positive."

The mammogram was replaced by a loose-leaf folder. Inside were a dozen studies comparing mastectomy to lumpectomy.

Julie wanted to save her life, but if she could, she wanted to save her breast too (if she had cancer). According to the studies in the folder, she could. All of them reported a similar survival rate for both operations: 70 to 75 percent of women with Julie's set of risk factors—premenopausal, with stage two invasive breast cancer—survived after a mastectomy, and 70 to 75 percent survived after a lumpectomy plus radiation.

Did Dr. Winters have a recommendation? Julie asked.

The surgeon shook his head. When the numbers were this close, he said, it was the patient's decision.

Julie looked at Peter.

"I'm happy either way."

Julie chose a lumpectomy.

Dr. Winter said he would schedule the surgery for Monday. His nurse would call Julie with the details.

Standing outside on the sidewalk in the brilliant winter sunlight, Julie could feel the fear lifting. Knowing her choices, knowing what she had to do, made her feel empowered, made her feel that she had regained control of her life, that she had wrested it back from cancer, from memory and family history.

Peter had a different reaction. For the first time he felt frightened. The shadow in the mammogram was small but it was tangible, substantial, not ephemeral, like Julie's words and feelings; it had mass and it had density and it could kill. It could kill Julie, and maybe someday it could kill Brittany. And, Peter thought, it could kill him, too; it could kill him by killing everything he loved.

· · ·

It snowed again on the morning of Julie's surgery. There was a thin layer of white frosting on the bedroom window when the Contes woke up at six.

"The roads are going to be terrible," Peter said. He was sitting up in the bed, looking out the window. He and Julie had to be at Albert Einstein Medical Center at eight.

Julie got up and walked over to the window. Jerusalem Road was a mess; the hill on Old Darlington Road would be even worse. She was glad Susan had decided to sleep over.

The baby-sitting date had been made the night of the Winters visit; Julie had called everyone as soon as she got home.

The only really hard call was the one to her father. Since his retirement, Bob Mackey's interests had narrowed to the Philadelphia Flyers, the local hockey team. "I'm glad you called me," he said when Julie told him about the surgery, then lapsed into silence.

"They're not even sure it's cancer, Dad," Julie said.

"Good."

Julie could hear Yvonne in the background. But Yvonne did not come to the phone.

"I have to go now, Dad."

Her father asked Julie where she was having the surgery.

"Einstein, Dad."

"What's your room number?"

"You don't get a room number until you're admitted, Dad."

"Then I'll ask at the desk," he said. "Someone there will know where you are."

Aunt Grace was upbeat. "You got it early," she said. "That's the important thing. They can cure it when you get it early. You did the right thing, Julie. Everything's going to be fine. I'm not worried at all."

Emily sounded upbeat, too. But Emily burst into tears when Julie hung up. Susan was more puzzled than tearful. Why did God keep sparing her? Susan wondered. No husband, no children. She was the perfect victim. It seemed unfair.

Lisa, who spoke to Julie from San Diego, cried in her hotel room, and she cried again an hour later in a little restaurant overlooking San Diego Bay. Lisa still remembers every detail of the day Julie called. She remembers that as she sat in her hotel room talking to Julie, a late afternoon breeze from the bay was blowing in, and outside in the hall, loud, slightly drunken male voices were shouting at each other in Spanish.

After she hung up, Lisa thought of something that Beth, Aunt Grace's daughter, had said to her after Jennifer got sick the first time. "That's three," Beth had declared, "Kay, Jennifer, and Gail." (Gail, a first cousin, had died of breast cancer ten years earlier.) Beth called it a terrible record but, she said, at least the laws of probability had been exhausted for a while. Everyone else in their generation would be safe now.

But Beth was wrong; the laws were still in play. No one was safe.

Susan came downstairs around seven. She asked about Brittany and Mark. Julie told her they were still asleep.

Mark had woken up at six for a feeding. But Julie did not mention that. She did not want to talk about her children this morning.

"Are you packed?" Susan was at the stove now, pouring a cup of coffee.

"I packed last night," Julie said.

Dr. Winters's nurse had said pack light, and Julie had complied. Her suitcase in the hall contained two nighties, lipstick, cologne, a copy of *Redbook* magazine, and a Salvation Kit: a vial of holy water, a relic—a bone chip from St. Francis of Assisi—and a handful of dirt from a Yugoslav holy site where the Blessed Mother was reputed to have made an appearance.

Colleen McGuillicudy, the friend who gave Julie the Salvation Kit, also provided instructions on its use. Before the lumpectomy, Colleen said, Julie was to pour the holy water on her breast, cover the water with dirt from the holy site, then place St. Francis's bone chip on top of the muddy mixture and say a prayer.

The ritual sounded a little nutty to Julie, but she did not think it was any nuttier than anything else that was going to happen to her today. Cut open in two places; a pie-shaped segment of breast tissue and tumor (maybe) scooped out of her breast; a string of lymph nodes cut from her armpit. Julie's postoperative treatment would be even nuttier. Toxic chemicals would be poured into her body, chemicals that would make her hair fall out, that would shut down her immune system, that would make her vomit and retch for days on end.

The Blessed Mother and St. Francis could argue that, like everything else in life, nuttiness is relative.

"Ready?" Peter already had his coat on. He was standing in the hall with the suitcase in his hand.

Julie kissed Susan good-bye, then walked out to the hall. "Ready," she said.

There was a red light at the Newtown Turnpike–Route 684 intersection. The car skidded slightly when Peter stopped. The road was slippery. The snow had turned to rain.

"Nervous?" Peter asked.

"Uh-huh. A little."

"It'll be all right."

"Hold my hand," Julie said.

Peter put his hand on top of Julie's and squeezed it gently.

The light changed and the car began to move.

Julie wondered what Peter was thinking. To date, his most expansive statement on the object in the mammogram had been: "We'll get through this, somehow." What was Peter feeling besides determined? Was he also feeling angry? afraid? sad? Did he ever feel like crying?

"Did you take anything to read?" Peter asked.

The Contes were on the expressway now. Albert Einstein Medical Center was at the next exit.

"Redbook."

A blue Tercel pulled into the next lane. Julie looked at the driver. She was about twenty-three or twenty-four and seemed preoccupied. Probably thinking about her boyfriend, Julie thought. The Tercel suddenly shot ahead of Peter, then cut abruptly into the lane in front of him.

"Jesus, did you see that?"

Julie could only see the back of the young woman's head now. She had thick, frizzy hair like Emily and Susan. Lisa and Jennifer had the straightest hair in the family. Julie was in the middle. Not too frizzy, not too straight. Middle sister, middle hair. Another car cut in front of Peter. The blue Tercel disappeared.

"Good-bye, Frizzy Hair. Have a nice day." How could Frizzy Hair not have a nice day, Julie thought. Frizzy Hair was going to an office; she was going to see her friends, call her boyfriend, order take-out Chinese for lunch.

Frizzy Hair does not know what a lucky girl she is today.

Before the surgery, Dr. Winters told Julie he would not remove her lymph nodes unless he found a tumor. That piece of intelligence turned out to be the tip-off.

"What did she have?"

The voice was coming from behind Julie, from behind her and away from her; it was coming from the other side of the recovery room.

"A lumpectomy with nodes," a different voice said.

The last word floated down, featherlike, through the layers of anesthetic and landed on top of Julie's drugged brain, where it set off a neural chain reaction: "Nodes . . . malignant . . . cancer. I have cancer."

Julie fell back to sleep.

When she woke up again, a man in a white coat was smiling at her.

No—three men in white coats were smiling at her. The trio had wonderful, lilting Indian accents. One man was a radiologist, the other two were oncologists. Or was it the other way around? Julie was not sure. She would have asked the doctors to tell her their specialties again, but she was vomiting into a bedpan now. Julie felt self-conscious at first, but then she realized that the doctors were there to visit her cancer, not her. They talked about the cancer's amazing properties and qualities, about its ability to create blood vessels out of nothing, to eat through bone. The doctors were putting their business cards on the nightstand when Julie fell asleep again.

Eric Lindros!

Someone was talking about Eric Lindros now. Someone was saying: "For my money, Lindros is the best forward in hockey."

Julie opened one eye.

It was her father.

He was sitting at the foot of the bed in a duck hat.

"Hey, you're awake!" Peter was also sitting at the foot of the bed.

"Uh-huh," Julie said.

Now another voice was telling Julie how good she looked for someone who had just had surgery. Julie opened the other eye. Hank Conte, Peter's father, was sitting at the foot of the bed, too.

Julie stared at the eager, hapless trio at the foot of the bed for a moment, then fell back to sleep.

The next time she woke up, her father and Hank Conte were gone. But there was a new visitor in the room. Dr. Winters. He gave Julie a big smile.

"It went very well. I was just telling Peter; you're as strong as a horse." More compliments. But somewhere in between "you'll be out of here in no time" and "I wish all my patients were like you," the phrase "a two-point-two-centimeter tumor" flew by. Julie only happened to hear it because she was looking for it.

"It's official, then?" she said. "I have cancer."

Dr. Winters nodded. "I'm afraid so. The tumor was malignant."

CHAPTER SIX

ONE DAY, A FEW WEEKS AFTER JULIE'S LUMPECTOMY, A SUBURBAN hospital ran an ad in the *Philadelphia Inquirer* for its High-Risk Cancer Patient Program. Underneath the headline, there was a line drawing of a woman's head and upper torso. Underneath the drawing, a series of bulleted points marched the reader's eye down to the bottom of the page. Emily, who was having breakfast, read each bulleted item carefully.

There was a telephone number after the last bullet. She picked up the phone and dialed the number.

A week later, Emily found herself in a classroom in one of the few remaining intact sections of Camden, New Jersey, a manufacturing town across the river from Philadelphia. A dozen other women of various ages were seated in metal chairs around her. The meeting was supposed to be an orientation, and for the first half hour it was. The head of the hospital's High-Risk Cancer Patient Program, a professorial, fiftyish woman named Dr. Arlene Lowenstein,* explained how the pro-

*Pseudonym

262

gram worked, how it assessed risk, and how it tailored a monitoring schedule to each participant's individual level of risk.

But when Dr. Lowenstein finished, the women began to talk among themselves, about themselves and about their families. For the next hour, the women talked about the dead and the dying and about their own fear of dying. They talked about lost breasts, lost hopes, lost mothers and aunts and sisters and cousins—and husbands. As the hour dragged on, Emily found it harder and harder to breathe. The pain in the room was like fire; it was devouring all the oxygen in the air.

One of the women at the meeting already had breast cancer. But she no longer had breasts. A serial double mastectomy had claimed both. The first breast was taken by disease, the second was offered up later in sacrifice. One good breast in exchange for a livable life. But the exchange had not worked. The cancer had metastasized anyway. The woman was dying now. Even as she sat there on the edge of her metal chair, Emily could see the cancer eating the life out of her, killing her. There was hardly anything left of her. The woman said she knew she could not save herself; it was too late for her now. But she was going to save her sister.

After this meeting, Emily decided that she would remain childless.

On a Saturday afternoon in early March, Peter called Arizona. He was not sure why he was calling Rick. But some nagging sense of guilt or obligation made him feel that Rick was owed a call. He already knew about Julie; Aunt Grace had told him in January. But Peter felt that one of them, he or Julie, ought to speak to Rick.

"I think it should be you," Julie said, when the subject of the call first came up. "You know how Rick can be."

Rick was out when Peter called at one. He left his number and a message on Rick's answering machine.

When Rick called back, Julie picked up the phone in the kitchen. "Hello?"

"Julie, is that you?"

"Rick, hi. How are you?"

"Julie, I'm so sorry for you."

Julie was too startled to say anything.

"It's just so terrible."

Julie took a deep breath. "It's okay, Rick. I've got a good prognosis. I'm going to be all right."

"I'm sorry, Julie. I know Jennifer would be heartbroken."

"The tumor was very small, Rick. They got it early."

"I'm so sorry," Rick said again.

Julie felt a wave of anger. Rick had her dead already. Another deep breath.

"Rick, how are the girls? How are Deidre and Melody doing?'

Later that night, Julie began to feel guilty. She had practically slammed the phone down after Rick finished describing Melody's school play. He must have sensed how eager she was to hang up. "I suppose I should have expected him to be fatalistic," Julie said. "After Jennifer and everything, how could he not be? Rick probably thinks every woman with breast cancer dies. But I'm not Jennifer, I'm me."

"Remember that," Peter told her.

A few days after the conversation with Rick, Julie began her journey through Cancerland. The first person she met there was Dr. Nathaniel Epstein* at Albert Einstein. "I think you'll like him," said the cheerful Dr. Winters when he recommended Epstein. But Julie did not like the short, bald, intense Dr. Epstein. He might be a tremendous oncologist, but he was too fond of statistics for Julie's taste. "Not Epstein," Julie told Peter after the visit.

Dr. Michael Allen,* Dr. Winters's next recommendation, was famous throughout the Einstein system; he had "the touch" with patients, Dr. Winters said. But Julie did not like him, either. He had a big-

*Pseudonym

ger office and a prettier secretary than Dr. Epstein, and he was less intense, but he shared Dr. Epstein's fondness for numbers; he also seemed in a tremendous hurry. He had the Contes in and out of his office in under fifteen minutes.

"Not Allen," Julie told Peter in the car.

Around this time, Julie discovered a new way to drive herself crazy. At night, lying in the dark, listening to the restless sputter of Peter's snore, she would visualize her cancer cells; she would imagine the cells emerging from hiding places in the fat and muscle tissues, imagine them multiplying and dividing; she would watch as one cell became two; two cells, four; four, eight; eight, sixteen; sixteen, thirty-two; thirty-two, sixty-four. On a bad night, Julie could have half a million new cancer cells by 2 A.M.

"I'm making myself crazy," she told Peter a few days after the visit to Dr. Allen.

Barbara Fowble was the next doctor on Julie's list. Dr. Fowble was at Fox Chase Cancer Center, which Julie liked. Fox Chase was one of the best cancer hospitals in the United States. It was also convenient. And Dr. Fowble was a woman, something else Julie liked. A woman might be more understanding and easier to talk to.

One wet Tuesday afternoon at the end of March, Julie descended into the subbasement of Fox Chase's main building, wove through a warren of cubicles, passed a storage room and a door with an exit sign over it, and stopped in front of a narrow rectangular office. Inside the office, a small, round, blond woman in an ankle-length white coat was sitting on a stool examining an X ray. The woman looked like a character in a storybook: the Queen of Hearts perched atop an oversized mushroom. Julie could not find a door to knock on. She rapped a fist on the door frame. The woman looked up and smiled.

Right away, Julie sensed that Dr. Fowble was different.

During her first few weeks in Cancerland, Julie had felt "objectified," reduced to a set of probabilities. "You have a 75 percent chance of living, Mrs. Conte, and a 25 percent chance of dying." Dr. Epstein,

Dr. Allen, all doctors who worked in Cancerland were decent and thoughtful, but no matter where they started or where they went, they always returned to the numbers and, in Julie's case, to three numbers in particular, to the 75 percent, the 25 percent, and to 2.2 centimeters, the circumference of her tumor.

Dr. Fowble was a physician who knew how to sound humane as well as smart. Which is to say, a physician who understood exactly where Julie's disease and her life intersected.

"You'll still be able to take care of your children and to work while you're on chemo," Dr. Fowble told Julie during their first meeting. "You'll feel nauseous sometimes, but you'll be able to manage."

No one else had mentioned that to Julie.

Dr. Fowble also reassured Julie about her choice to have a lumpectomy.

A few nights earlier, in between counting her new cancer cells, Julie had had a very bad few minutes about the lumpectomy. I made a mistake, she thought. I made the wrong choice and now I'm going to die because of it. I should have had a mastectomy.

"No, you made the right choice," Dr. Fowble told her now. "A lumpectomy was the appropriate surgery in your case."

"Definitely, Fowble," Julie told Peter that night.

But there was a complication. At Fox Chase, as at other cancer centers, two treatment modalities, radiation and chemotherapy, are used against breast cancer. Dr. Fowble was a radiation oncologist; Julie would need a medical oncologist to administer chemotherapy. The medical oncologist Dr. Fowble usually worked with was Dr. Lori Goldstein. So ten days later, Julie and Peter made a second visit to Fox Chase.

Dr. Goldstein's office was tucked away in a corner of a laboratory on the second floor. The office was even smaller than Dr. Fowble's, but it had a wonderful view. It looked out on a lovely little park full of intersecting walkways, rolling hills, and spruce and birch trees. Warm April sunlight was flooding through a window when the Contes arrived at noon for Julie's appointment.

"Mr. and Mrs. Conte?"

Julie nodded.

Dr. Goldstein, who was about Julie's age, stood up and walked over to greet them.

"I'm sorry, my hands are very cold." She rubbed a hand against her coat, then offered it to Julie.

"Come in," Dr. Goldstein said.

Julie took the seat by the window. People were sitting in the park. Hospital staff, probably. Most of the men had their sport jackets off and their shirt collars unbuttoned. Spring, finally!

Dr. Goldstein sat down.

A secretary came into the office and handed her a document. The oncologist flipped through it quickly, then looked at Julie.

"This is a protocol for a new study," she said. "It's for women like you, Julie: early stage disease, but with a high relapse risk." Dr. Goldstein handed Julie the protocol. "I'd like you to take it home and read it. It will explain how the study works. I think you'd be a good candidate for it."

Julie took the protocol and looked over at Peter. He seemed as surprised as she was by the sales pitch. The meeting had just begun.

"I thought we were going to talk about treatment today," he said.

"I can treat Julie with standard therapy," Dr. Goldstein said. "But I really think Julie would benefit from this study. I would recommend participation."

Julie opened the protocol and flipped through it. Dr. Goldstein was staring at her when she looked up again.

"I'd really urge you to consider it, Julie. You're node negative and that's very good. I think you'd really benefit from this protocol."

Julie said she and Peter would discuss the study and let Dr. Goldstein know.

"What did you think of her?" Julie asked when she and Peter were in the hall.

"It's your call," Peter said.

"They're a package," Julie said. "If I want Fowble, I have to take Goldstein."

Nothing was ever simple in Cancerland.

In the car, Julie took the protocol out of her bag and opened it.

The three study drugs, Adriamycin, Cytoxan (cyclophosphamide), and tamoxifen, were familiar to her; they were familiar to almost anyone who worked in a hospital. Tamoxifen, the newest of the drugs, was ten years old. But the study was going to use two of the study agents, Adriamycin and Cytoxan, in a novel way.

Preliminary evidence indicated that at very high dose levels, the two agents had significantly greater cancer-killing power. SWOG 9313, was going to test this proposition as well as the safety of giving high doses of highly toxic Adriamycin and Cytoxan.

SWOG study 9313 had another objective. It would try to answer a question oncologists had been debating for a decade: Did tamoxifen, an antiestrogen agent, reduce the risk of relapse from breast cancer?

Julie scanned the table of contents. Side effects and adverse reactions were described on page forty-one. She opened to page forty-one. The first side effect described was death, though the word itself was not used. In a protocol, no one actually dies; they suffer a fatality or fatal incident. The reference to death was in a paragraph headlined "High-Dose Therapy." The paragraph began:

"Higher-dose therapy, such as the treatment you may receive in this study, is associated with a range of increased toxicities compared to standard therapy. Other toxicities that could occur later might also be life-threatening, even fatal."

On the next page, Julie found a description of each individual test drug's side effects.

According to the protocol, Adriamycin could produce nausea, vomiting, decreased white blood cell count, skin discoloration, mouth sores, fever, chills, facial flushing, swollen eyelids, heart failure, acute leukemia, red urine, and baldness, including genital baldness.

Cytoxan (also known as cyclophosphamide), the next drug described, did everything that Adriamycin did, as well as a few things Adriamycin did not do, such as scar the lungs and induce sterility in both sexes.

However, tamoxifen, the third drug in the trial, was the real star of the adverse-reactions section. Nearly two pages were required to describe all the things tamoxifen could do to the human body. Its side effects included depression, leg cramps, gastrointestinal malignancies, confusion, vaginal bleeding, uterine cancer, polyps, and genital itching.

Julie knew that even the rarest adverse reactions had to be included in a study protocol; still . . .

"What do you think?" Peter said. They were at the Route 684–Newton Turnpike intersection now. Almost home.

"I don't know," Julie said. "The protocol sounds scary."

"Hold still, honey."

Brittany shook her head and giggled.

It was the morning after the Goldstein visit and Julie was in the living room dressing Brittany for day care.

"I won't put the bow in your hair if you're a bad girl."

Brittany pouted but she stopped shaking her head.

There was a clip under the bow. Julie slipped the clip underneath a clump of hair, then leaned back and smiled.

"Oh, don't you look like a pretty girl. Do you want to see how pretty you look?"

"Uh-huh." Brittany was suddenly beaming.

There was a mirror on the medicine cabinet door. Julie took Brittany into the hall bathroom, lifted her onto the toilet seat, and turned the cabinet door toward her.

"Pretty girl," Julie said.

"Pretty Brittany," Brittany said.

Peter would be able to figure out Mark on his own. But he did not know how to attach a hair bow properly or how to brush hair so that it shone, or how to dress a doll, or how to buy makeup, or how to explain what happens when you get your period, or what makes a boy cute. Julie would have to make a list of things he would need to learn about raising a girl . . . just in case.

Peter might remarry, of course. At night, in between watching her cancer cells multiply and divide, Julie had considered at some length the possibility of Peter's remarrying. But he might marry someone who was so wrapped up in herself and her own children—now there was another novel thought, Peter having children with someone else—that she would ignore Brittany. It would be up to Peter to look after her, and Julie would have to teach . . .

"Mommy?"

Brittany was pointing a finger at Julie's face. Julie touched her cheek. It was wet. Oh shit, she thought, I'm crying.

"Honey, go outside and wait for Mommy. I'll be out in a minute."

After Brittany left, Julie looked in the mirror. Her makeup was streaky. She took a bottle of blush from the medicine cabinet and unscrewed the top.

"Mommy?" Brittany was standing outside the bathroom door.

"I'm coming, hon. I'll be out in a sec."

Julie dabbed on the blush and quickly put the bottle back in the cabinet. She checked herself in the mirror. There, normal again. Brittany was standing at the front door when Julie walked out of the bathroom.

"Ready, baby?"

Brittany smiled and pointed to herself. "Pretty Brittany," she said again.

That night, Julie told Peter she had decided to participate in the study.

CHAPTER SEVEN

THE MEDIA OFTEN MAKE DRUG RESEARCH SOUND AS SIMPLE AS A, B, C: Doctor A discovers drug B, and disease C is conquered, and everyone lives happily ever after.

In the case of a home-run drug like insulin or penicillin, in the case of a drug that is both safe and effective, the process is almost that simple. But in breast cancer—in all cancers—there are no home-run drugs.

Pretty good drugs require a second, unglamorous level of research—strategy research. Strategy research focuses on usage. How do you use a group of imperfect drugs in a way that allows the drugs to save the maximum number of human lives, despite their shortcomings?

Over the last three decades, the answer for breast cancer, indeed for all cancers, has been combination chemotherapy. In twos and threes, pretty good drugs can compensate for one another's weaknesses and flaws. Drug B will do what drug A cannot do and drug C will do what drug B cannot do.

The idea of using cancer drugs together is now so widely accepted, it sounds almost commonsensical. But in the early 1970s, many people thought that combining highly toxic drugs was crazy. The strategy might be worth trying in women who had run out of hope and luck, who would die from their disease even if the toxic drugs did not kill them. But it was too dangerous to use in women with less advanced breast cancer. However, supporters of the strategy believed that this was precisely the population who would benefit most from combination chemotherapy. In relatively healthy women, the strategy might not just slow the progress of the disease, it might save lives.

The National Cancer Institute was ambivalent. Though it had approved a single-agent study in the 1970s, it remained opposed to using more toxic two- and three-drug combinations against less advanced disease. So this American idea had to be tested first in Italy. In 1975, Giovanni Bonadonna of the Milan Institute tested a regimen of three drugs, CMF—cyclophosphamide, methotrexate, and 5-fluorouracil—in a group of women with less advanced disease.

The Bonadonna study, which found that CMF measurably decreased the incidence of relapse, created a new standard of breast cancer care: surgery, now often a less severe lumpectomy, radiation for local disease (i.e., the cancer in the breast); and postoperative combination chemotherapy for systemic disease, for the metastasizing cells in the blood. However, in the early 1980s, one group of patients still remained outside the chemotherapy umbrella: women with no node involvement, women with small tumors, women like Julie.

No one thought that these patients needed anything more than what they were already getting—the traditional therapies of surgery and radiation.

In the mid-1980s, however, a new study made everyone think again.

It showed that node-positive subjects—which is to say, women with more advanced cancers—fared better with the addition of chemotherapy than node-negative women, women with less advanced cancers, who were treated with surgery and radiation alone. The ratio of relapse was startling: 5 percent versus 12 percent.

In the late 1980s, enough research was available to define what might be called the high-risk–low-risk woman. Essentially, she was Julie. She was node negative, had a tumor between 2 and 5 centimeters, and often, estrogen-receptor negative cancer cells. This last characteristic is considered an additional risk factor, because as cancer cells progress toward malignancy, they lose the characteristics of normal breast cells, like receptor sites.

In 1988, the National Cancer Institute issued a special treatment advisory on the high-risk–low-risk woman. The agency said that, henceforth, she should also receive combination chemotherapy postsurgically.

The advisory has made some difference, but not enough.

"Here are these women with little tiny tumors in their breast, and ten years later 25 percent of them are dead," says Dr. Barbara Fowble, Julie's radiologist. "That's shocking."

The stated goal of SWOG 9313 is to reduce the death rate among high-risk–low-risk women by a third. But to achieve the goal, SWOG's designers, Dr. C. Kent Osborne of the University of Texas and Dr. Charles Haskell of UCLA, are taking a gamble.

SWOG is testing a new and controversial high-dose sequential strategy.

In the spring of 1980, Canadian oncologist William Hryniuk was a very excited man. Often, you can make breast cancer go away the first time, but a second disappearance is hard to produce, even a temporary one. The remission rate among relapse patients is abysmally low.

What Dr. Hryniuk noticed in the spring of 1980 was a remission rate of 76 percent among relapse patients at McMasters University in Hamilton, Ontario. "I couldn't believe it," says the researcher. "It seemed too good to be true." But Dr. Hryniuk was also puzzled. The

McMasters patients were on the same drug regimen—a souped-up version of CMF—as were metastatic patients everywhere else. Why was CMF producing a miracle in the middle of Canada and nowhere else? Dr. Hryniuk compared the treatment records of the patients who were in remission against those who were not.

Only one difference emerged. Patients in the remission group got the same amount of chemotherapy, but they received the CMF regimen over a shorter period of time. What this suggested was so simple, at first Dr. Hryniuk could not believe it: You could enhance the cancer-killing power of a drug simply by giving the drug over shorter intervals of time.

The Hryniuk discovery quickly acquired a name, dose intensity, and an application. Since the mid-1980s, it has been used in a treatment for the very sick—bone marrow transplant recipients. But in the early 1990s several investigators began to argue that dose intensity could have another application; it might have a role to play in the treatment of the less sick, in women like Julie.

But as with combination chemotherapy a generation earlier, the strategy created a risk/benefit problem. Giving powerful drugs at frequent intervals not only makes it easier for those drugs to penetrate cancer cells—the reason that giving a drug over a shorter period enhances its potency—it also increases the drug's toxicity. Existing therapies could already cure three-quarters of high risk–low risk women. Was it ethical to expose this group, this 75 percent of women who were going to live anyway, to an increased risk of heart disease and leukemia in order to try to save some of the women who would die if treated conventionally?

To this godlike question, a new drug called G-CSF, which speeds up the recovery time of a chemo-ravaged immune system, offered a partial answer. But like everything else in the cancer medicine cabinet, G-CSF is only a pretty good drug. To create an acceptable risk level for women like Julie, the combination-chemo strategy—the foundation of modern cancer therapy—would have to be abandoned. Chemo agents would have to be given one after the other, instead of together. But this sequential strategy creates its own risk.

There are several different kinds of cancer cells. Giving drug A alone will allow you to give A at a higher dose and more frequently. But while you're killing A-vulnerable cancer cells, drug B-vulnerable cells will continue to grow unmolested, and this population could be so large by the time you finish killing the A cells that no amount of drug B will be able to wipe it out—at least, no amount a human being can take and still be alive the next day.

However, in the 1980s Dr. Larry Norton of Memorial Sloan-Kettering Hospital in New York said that, in some cases, it was safe to abandon the combination strategy, because you really do not have to worry about the B-vulnerable cancer cells, at least not right away.

Dr. Norton's answer to the B problem grew out of an encounter he had had in the summer of 1973 with a patient he never expected to see again.

"I was sure I had cured the man a year earlier," says Dr. Norton.

But now the young man was sick again. His Hodgkin's disease had come back. How could a cured cancer return?

Dr. Norton, who sees the world through numbers, sat down with a pencil and paper and did some calculations. He looked at how the Hodgkin's patient had responded to treatment and he looked at the data on tumor growth, which, in the early seventies, was thought to be exponential: one cell becomes two, two become four, four become eight, etc. When the researcher put the two sets of numbers together, they predicted a cure for the patient.

So why had the young man relapsed?

Dr. Norton concluded that either the patient's cancer had not shrunk as quickly as the data on his medical record indicated (and Norton remembered) or tumor growth was not exponential.

Norton began to search through the literature on tumor development. Eventually, the search led him back to the nineteenth century and to Benjamin Gompertz, a British mathematician who developed a new theory of population growth. The theory, which was published in an 1825 issue of the *Philosophical Transactions of the Royal Society*, had one of those grandiloquent Victorian titles, "On the Nature of the Function Expressive of the Law of Human Mortality," and it is probably the single best thing that ever happened to the insurance industry.

Gompertz said that human populations grow in a very predictable way. At the beginning, when a population is new, when everyone is young and reproducing, there is a ferocious burst of growth, exponential-like growth. Later, as people age, growth flags, and as the people begin to die off, growth stops completely.

Actuaries were the first to realize that Gompertz's ideas had a practical value. If you could accurately predict how long a given population would live, you could make a lot of money selling life insurance to members of the population. By the time Johns Hopkins biologist Charles Windsor wrote about Gompertz in the early 1930s, it was clear that other things also grew according to the Gompertzian curve, including the shell of the razor clam and the rat. In the 1960s, Dr. Anna Laird, a National Cancer Institute investigator, discovered that tumor growth also is Gompertzian.

When Dr. Norton came across the Laird paper, he redid his calculations for the Hodgkin's patient based on Gompertzian tumor growth patterns. This time the numbers predicted a relapse.

Dr. Norton thinks that some version of the Gompertz curve may turn out to be a universal principle. "I think one day we might discover that everything, rocks, dust balls, tumors, human populations, clam shells, everything grows the same way: fast, then slow, then not at all." One corollary of Gompertz's theory about growth is that everything also has a growth limit, a limit beyond which the thing cannot grow. In the case of a tumor, Dr. Norton thinks the limit may be two or three liters, approximately the size of a small child. If the body could sustain it, that's how large some tumors would become.

The high-dose sequential strategy grew out of Norton's work on Gompertzian tumor growth. The researcher found that tumor growth is uneven—fast, then slow—because cancer cells replicate at different rates. Fast breeders, which are often highly malignant, provide the explosive exponential-like growth at the beginning of the tumor life cycle. But fast breeders are usually in a minority in a tumor; at a certain point, slower-breeding B cells have to start making a contribution, and as they do, tumor growth slows.

The sequential strategy, a Norton creation, says that since fast-breeding A cancer cells pose the most urgent danger, attack them first with a very high dose of the drug they are most vulnerable to. This will mean granting slow-breeding B cells a temporary stay of execution. It would be too toxic to use a second drug. But the sequential strategy says that this is safe, because B cells breed slowly.

Among the many things that will be clearer after the completion of SWOG 9313 is whether or not the high-dose sequential strategy is right about B cells.

One warm evening in May 1992, the Breast Committee of the Southwest Oncology Group gathered in a hotel conference room in San Antonio, Texas, to make an important decision.

Node-negative breast cancer patients are an important priority for SWOG, which is a research consortium of cancer institutions in the West and Southwest. SWOG 8897, the consortium's current study for these women, who, like Julie, tend to be young, would end in early 1993. That night, the committee had to decide what its member institutions would do to help them next.

One committee member, the chairman, C. Kent Osborne of the University of Texas, proposed a daring and innovative idea.

Dr. Osborne suggested a study that would use two old chemo warhorses, Adriamycin and Cytoxan, but in a new way, a way that would combine Dr. Hryniuk's ideas about frequency and Dr. Norton's ideas about potency and tumor growth. Dr. Osborne thought that, used correctly, the two strategies might turn two pretty good drugs into two much better drugs.

The trial Dr. Osborne outlined to the committee that night would be relatively short, eighteen weeks, and both arms would get Adriamycin and Cytoxan in the same doses. But whereas women in the control group would get the drugs in the traditional combination fashion over the eighteen weeks, patients in the experimental arm would get a treatment schedule based on Dr. Hryniuk's ideas about dose intensity. The experimental arm would get twelve weeks of Adriamycin at a high dose instead of eighteen weeks at a traditional dose, and six weeks of Cytoxan at a high dose instead of eighteen weeks at the traditional dose.

Dr. Norton's influence was evident in Dr. Osborne's choice of a first drug for the experimental arm. In theory, an 81-milligram-per-treatment dose of Adriamycin, generally considered the best breast cancer drug, should be enough to obliterate all fast-breeding, often hypermalignant A cells.

SWOG 9313 would grant slow-breeding B cancer cells an extra twelve weeks of life. But then they would be attacked with very large doses of Cytoxan.

G-CSF would be used to offset toxicity problems.

Dr. Osborne also suggested that the study examine whether tamoxifen had a prophylactic effect on breast cancer. (Two years later, another study would find that it did.)

UCLA oncologist Charles Haskell, a member of the SWOG Breast Committee, remembers that, despite some concerns about toxicity, Dr. Osborne's ideas for what became 9313 got a very positive reception at the San Antonio meeting. "Everyone realized that if the strategy worked we could cut the death rate among low-risk women by 30 percent," Dr. Haskell says.

Everyone also realized that to conclusively demonstrate a 30 percent decline in a 25 to 30 percent death rate—9313's goal—the study would need to be very large. SWOG would have to recruit 3,000 women, with zero to three nodes and tumors between 2 and 5 centimeters.

Even though two other research consortiums, the Eastern Cooperative Oncology Group (Fox Chase is a member) and the North Center Cancer Treatment Group, agreed to contribute patients, it would take nearly three years to launch SWOG 9313. Indeed, when Julie and Peter visited Dr. Goldstein in April 1995, a copy of the trial protocol had just arrived on her desk. Julie was to become the first Fox Chase patient to enter the trial.

In late April, the ECOG computer tracking 9313 patients assigned her to Arm B, the treatment arm. Julie would receive the high-dose therapy.

CHAPTER EIGHT

THE PHYSICAL MECHANICS OF CHEMOTHERAPY ARE SIMPLE. ALL YOU need is a plastic bag, a pole, a rubber catheter, a chair, and a drug. But, of course, the bag is not just a bag, the chair is not just a chair, the drug is not just a drug. So the emotional mechanics of the treatment are more complex.

Julie was hoping that her experience as a medical professional would protect her. She had been in and out of the infusion room at St. Monica's dozens of times. She already knew what the paraphernalia of chemo looked like—the poles and bags and the liquid inside the bags. That experience had to be an advantage.

Julie also was hoping to get some help from the infusion center at Fox Chase. The nice thing about the center was that it seemed designed *not* to remind you of where you were or what you were doing there. The reception area, oak paneled with recessed lighting, looked like a law office, the infusion room like a beauty salon, or maybe an air-port waiting lounge, but it had a pleasant view. On summer afternoons,

Julie could sit in one of the chairs near the monitoring station and look out the window at the lovely little park in the center of the hospital.

"I like it here," she told Peter the day they toured the center. "I feel comfortable."

Julie would be very nervous on her first day of treatment, too nervous to deal with all the things that can go wrong in a hospital. But a nurse in Dr. Goldstein's office had assured her that the staff at the center would take care of everything. All Julie had to do was show up. However, the nurse failed to take two things into account. Julie was the first Fox Chase patient on 9313 and the chemo doses in 9313 were unusually large.

"Sheila, I need you. Could you come here, please?"

The nurse at the reception desk had just punched Julie's protocol number into a computer. Now she was crouched in front of a screen studying a row of orange numbers.

A second nurse appeared from behind the wood-paneled wall.

Nurse One pointed a worried finger at the numbers. "Have you ever seen doses like this before?"

Nurse Two looked at the screen. "Oh, my God, enormous, aren't they? Look." Now Nurse Two was pointing at the screen. "She's supposed to get another treatment tomorrow. I never heard of that. Back-to-back chemo."

Nurse One stood up and walked over to Julie. "I'm sorry, Mrs. Conte. I'm going to have call Dr. Goldstein's office. This is a new study. No one here is familiar with it."

Dr. Goldstein was on vacation.

"What about Patty?" Nurse Two said. She was still crouched in front of the computer screen. "Patty knows all the breast cancer protocols."

Patty was on an early lunch. Nurse One turned to Julie again. "I'm afraid we're going to have to do a little more checking, Mrs. Conte. The doses on your treatment schedule are very large. It's for your own safety. You understand."

Julie said she understood.

"No one is familiar with the study?" Aunt Grace exclaimed when Julie returned to the waiting area. "How can that be?" Grace had insisted on accompanying Peter and Julie this morning.

"Apparently, it's a brand-new study," Julie said, and sat down in the chair next to Grace to wait.

"Really," Grace said. "The staff should know better."

An hour later, Patty still had not returned from lunch. Grace looked at her watch. "Twelve-forty. We got here at eleven. This is ridiculous." The more agitated Grace got, the more she sounded like Margaret Thatcher. She stood up. "I'm going to see what's going on."

"Can I help you?" Nurse One said when Grace walked over to the desk.

"We've been waiting for nearly two hours, nurse. Do you have any more information on my niece's protocol?" Grace pointed at Julie.

"I'm sorry, ma'am, we're still checking."

"This is extraordinary." Grace was in a state now. Julie could tell. "I picked Fox Chase for my niece because I thought it would be an easier experience for her than Penn. She's a very sensitive girl . . ."

Peter looked at Julie.

Julie sighed.

Ten minutes later, a new nurse appeared at the reception desk. It was Patty; she was back from lunch. Julie could hear Patty talking to nurses One and Two. She was telling them that SWOG 9313 was a new breast cancer protocol. When she finished at the desk, Patty came into the waiting room. She was short and blond and had a sweet-tough Irish face. "Are you Mrs. Conte?" she asked Julie.

"Yes," Julie said.

"I'm sorry. We're usually more efficient than this. We'll be ready for you in a few minutes. If you want, you can pick up your G-CSF from the pharmacy while you're waiting."

Julie asked what G-CSF was.

Patty looked surprised. "No one told you about G-CSF?"

"I'm sure they did and I forgot," Julie said. No one had mentioned the drug to her.

"G-CSF keeps your white blood cell count up," Patty said. "You have to give yourself a shot five days after each chemo session. You do it right here." Patty pointed to a spot just above her navel. "In the stomach."

Julie must have looked horrified.

"It's not as bad as it sounds." Patty bent down and put a hand on Julie's shoulder. "All you feel is a little pinch when the needle goes in."

Nurse One came into the waiting room. "We're ready for you now, Mrs. Conte."

Patty squeezed Julie's shoulder. "Good luck," she said.

Julie felt underdressed when she walked into the infusion room. Everyone else had a hat on. Everywhere she looked she saw baseball caps and turbans, berets and skullcaps and scarfs.

"Here you are, Mrs. Conte."

Nurse One was standing in front of a chair near the monitoring desk. The ostrich-neck metal pole next to the chair already had a plastic bag on it. The nurse attached a catheter to the IV tubing at the bottom of the bag, then asked Julie to open her blouse.

"I want to check your port," the nurse said.

Most people have a small tubal-shaped port implanted in the chest before chemo so they will not have to take the drug intravenously (through the veins). But Julie, the big chemo expert, had forgotten about the port.

"I'm sorry, I don't have a port," she told the nurse.

The nurse started to explain why a port was important.

"I know why I need one," Julie said. "I just forgot, in the rush, you know with everything. Stupid me."

"Do you want to wait and get the port implanted first? I think that would be better."

"No," Julie said. "I want to start now."

Nurse One looked wary. "I'm going to have to put the drug into your vein, Mrs. Conte. I haven't done a vein in a while."

"Please, I just want to start," Julie said.

"Okay, I'll have to get a needle at the monitoring station." Julie had her blouse sleeve rolled up when the nurse came back. The nurse took Julie's arm and began to probe the soft inner flesh of the forearm for a vein.

"Oh shoot, I'm sorry," the nurse said. "I'll have to get another needle."

Julie heard the catheter drop on the floor but she did not see it. She was concentrating all her attention on a ceiling light directly overhead. It was light number eight in a row of thirteen recessed lights. There were three other rows in the ceiling and each row had exactly thirteen lights.

A moment later, Julie felt a finger probing her arm again. The nurse's gestures were tentative, uncertain. She must be very nervous, Julie thought. Light number eight was developing a halo. "Ouch." The nurse got the needle in this time. The halo was expanding, getting bigger, fatter. Points of light were flashing out from the halo. The points were becoming blinding. Julie could not see anymore.

The nurse was talking now. "Are you all right? Did I hurt you, Mrs. Conte? I'm sorry. Let me get you a Kleenex. You're crying."

Colleen McGuillicudy, one of Julie's friends at work, has a Rosie O'Donnell chin, Duchess of York freckles, a low center of gravity, glorious red hair, and a profound sense of religiosity, though some people in the public affairs department at St. Monica's consider Colleen's religiosity more weird than profound. Colleen talks about God, and especially about the Blessed Mother, in a very personal way. Indeed, sometimes, listening to Colleen talk about the Virgin Mary, Julie can almost see the two of them sitting together in the McGuillicudys' living room watching *Oprah* and swapping dieting tips.

Julie has always been very much of two minds about Colleen's religiosity, but after she got sick, one of those minds became a believer in heavenly messengers. This mind, which Julie thought of as her spiritual mind, believed that the tumor would still be in her breast, still growing and spreading but for the bolt of breastbone pain Jennifer sent down from heaven on January 2. Julie's spiritual mind also believed that if God worked through Jennifer, He might also work through other heavenly messengers, including, perhaps, Colleen. Which is how sweet, funny, neurotic Colleen became Julie's guardian angel. Sort of.

Colleen was the inspiration for the religious ritual that preceded the lumpectomy. Colleen supplied the holy water, the St. Francis relic, the dirt from the holy site, and the instructions on how to use them. She was also the inspiration for Julie's visit to the grave site of Blessed Catherine Drexel, founder of the Sisters of the Blessed Sacrament and currently Philadelphia's only candidate for sainthood.

The Blessed Catherine inspiration came to Colleen one muggy morning a week after Julie's first chemo. Colleen said a visit to the grave site would secure Blessed Catherine's personal support for a cure. "Jennifer and Blessed Catherine can visit God together and talk to him about you," Colleen said.

Julie thought the odds of Jennifer and Blessed Catherine buttonholing God on her behalf were approximately .000001 to 1. But then, Julie's spiritual mind reminded her that the chances of discovering a malignant tumor in your breast a week after your sister died of breast cancer were probably .00000001 to 1.

Julie asked Colleen where Blessed Catherine's grave was.

"Bensalem."

Poor Blessed Catherine, Julie thought. Bensalem had even more Wawas and Arby's than Route 684.

"We can be there in twenty minutes," Colleen said. "Why don't we go today at lunch."

Julie paused for a moment, then said all right, lunch, today; it was fine with her.

. . .

The Blessed Catherine Drexel grave site is on the grounds of St. Elizabeth's convent, a few miles from Bensalem's central shopping district. You approach the convent grounds through an alley of auto body repair shops and pizzerias and cheap flower shops. After the last flower shop, there is a handsome gray stone gate. After the gate, another world: the postmodern honky-tonk of Bensalem gives way to the redemptive dreams of the nineteenth-century German and Irish immigrants who built the convent. There are acres of stately green lawn, swirling gravel roads, and faintly Gothic sandstone buildings shaded by poplar and willow trees.

"Blessed Catherine's grave is in the chapel," Colleen said as she pulled into the parking lot. Julie looked around. No other cars, no other petitioners. Suddenly she and Colleen had become the last two people on earth. When the car stopped, Julie opened her purse and took out a veil. The veil, black with a frilly kind of lace, was a get-well present from a girl at work. Julie turned the rearview mirror toward her, fiddled with the veil for a moment, then got out of the car and walked across the empty parking lot. The crunch of her Reeboks on the gravel sounded loud in the stillness.

Blessed Catherine's final resting place was an elevated gray-black marble tomb in the center of a small chapel attached to St. Elizabeth's convent. Julie and Colleen walked through an archway into the chapel; at the tomb, they knelt and made the sign of the cross.

"Touch her," Colleen whispered.

Julie looked at Colleen.

Colleen pointed to the marble tomb. "Go ahead. Touch."

Julie put her hand on top of the marble. It felt cool and moist.

Julie looked at Colleen again.

"Now say: 'Blessed Catherine Drexel.' Call her. Say 'Blessed Catherine' out loud."

Julie felt a little embarrassed. She turned around. The chapel was still empty. "Blessed Catherine," Julie said. Her voice made an echo.

"Now put your hand on your breast. Where the tumor was."

Boom. Another echo. This one tremendous. Julie looked at Colleen again.

"My purse fell," Colleen said.

Julie touched the area of her breast where the tumor had been. It was still sore from the surgery.

"Now ask Catherine to intercede for you."

"Out loud?" Julie asked.

"You can talk to her any way you want," Colleen said.

Julie prayed for a minute or two, then stood up and made the sign of the cross again.

The parking lot felt very hot after the cool of the chapel. Julie took her veil off and put it in her purse. She had hoped to be inspired by the visit, but all she felt now was deflated, deflated and a little silly. Where did Colleen get these rituals?

"You okay?" Colleen asked.

Julie nodded and opened the car door.

After Colleen got in, she opened her purse. "Here, I have something for you." Colleen took a card out of her purse and handed it to Julie.

The front of the card was blank; Julie turned it over. On the back, there were a few lines of what looked like a poem. A note at the top of the card said that the author of the lines, a Jewish woman, was killed during the Warsaw Ghetto uprising. A few weeks before her death, the woman had written:

> *I believe in sun, even when there is no sun.*
> *I believe in happiness, even when there is no laughter.*
> *I believe in God, even when He is silent.*

Dr. Goldstein had on slipper-shaped midnight blue shoes this morning. The silver piping around the toes was nifty. Julie liked the little-girl white socks above the slipper shoes, too. They looked like silk, but Julie was sitting too far away to tell for sure. Above the socks, Julie saw leg, then a hint of patterned skirt, then a sea of crisp, Alaskan white. Dr. Goldstein had her medical coat buttoned up this morning.

Julie herself looked like an army recruit. An army recruit or Uncle Fester, she could not make up her mind which, when she looked at herself in the bathroom mirror. The Uncle Fester haircut was a preemptive strike. Julie reasoned that the less hair she had to lose, the less bad she would feel about losing it. But in the presence of the seriously chic Dr. Goldstein, the Uncle Fester haircut made Julie feel self-conscious.

The oncologist opened a manila folder and spoke. "To answer your question, hair loss usually begins after the second Adriamycin treatment." Julie had just asked when she would start to go bald.

Dr. Goldstein had wonderful hair. It was thick and black and shiny and a little fuzzy, too. Julie was developing a theory about Dr. Goldstein. She was actually rather nice; the formality, the stiffness was a ruse, a strategy to offset her youth, which probably worried some patients.

Dr. Goldstein's prediction about the hair loss was accurate. A few days after her second treatment, Julie noticed a bald spot while she was getting dressed for work. It was on the left side of her head about three inches above the ear. Julie leaned into the bathroom mirror. Where there used to be thick, fuzzy brown hair, there was now an ugly scaly red spot. Julie's gaze dropped a few inches. Oh God, there was also a bald spot on her left eyebrow. It looked like army ants had eaten their way though the middle of the brow. Julie pulled down her panties. Thank God! Her pubic hair had not started to fall out yet.

Dr. Goldstein also told Julie that she would feel some nausea after the first Adriamycin, but would not become sick until after the second. This prediction was also accurate, if a bit incomplete. Julie had not expected the nausea to come on so abruptly. One minute she and the nurses were chatting about Julie's new port; the next, Julie's stomach was in her throat. Lisa, the designated companion for the day, got Julie to the ladies' room just in time.

"Maybe we should get some help in?" Peter said that night. "You can't work, take care of the kids, and have chemo."

Julie said yes she could. She could do everything she needed to do.

What Julie could and should do was becoming a source of contention between her and Peter. What Peter really wanted was for Julie to take a leave of absence, to stop working for the duration of the chemo. Failing that, he wanted to bring in someone three or four days a week to help at home.

This was the second time Peter had suggested help, the second time Julie had said no.

"You know you don't have to prove how strong you are," Peter told her.

Julie said she was not trying to prove anything. She would just rather be busy. Busy kept her mind off the cancer.

Peter was skeptical.

Kay Mackey was putting up storm windows six months before her death. Her daughters wanted to be just as strong. You worked until you dropped and you never complained. The World According to the Mackey Women.

The next morning when Julie came down for breakfast, Peter was making lunch for Mark and Brittany. "I'll take the kids to day care," he said. Over the next few weeks, Peter quietly assumed other maternal duties. Julie appreciated the help, but she had some trouble accepting it. Peter was a dutiful but unimaginative mother. Julie liked Brittany in blue OshKoshes, not in gray, and always trimmed the crusts from her sandwiches; Peter liked whatever clothes were clean and whatever bread was handy, crusts or no crusts.

At a barbecue one Saturday, Julie tried to pump Peter's sister Carol for information. Had Peter spoken to her "about . . ." no word immediately leapt to mind, so Julie used the all-purpose "everything."

"Sort of," Carol said warily.

Julie asked what "sort of" meant.

"I know you're going to be fine, Julie," Carol said. "I want you to know that."

Julie said she knew that. "What did Peter say?"

The week before, Carol and her mother had been talking about how Peter would need help if anything happened. "Peter overheard us. And he was like, 'Yeah, I will need help.'"

"Did he say anything else?"

Carol looked wary again. "He doesn't know whether he'd keep the house if anything happened."

"So. You don't know whether you'll keep the house if anything happens to me?" Julie said that night.

Peter put down his paper. "Who said that?"

"You said that. Carol told me this afternoon."

"I don't remember saying anything about the house."

"Well, you did," Julie insisted.

Peter winced. "Oh God, I was just talking. It doesn't mean anything. You're going to be fine, Julie. I'm sure of it."

"You sound like your sister."

"Julie, I'm sorry."

Julie was still angry, but she made herself stop.

"You have to be considerate to Peter," Aunt Grace had told her. "He is carrying a tremendous burden. You have to give him some breathing space. You have to be kind to him."

Grace was right. Peter was carrying an awful burden. And it was aging him. Julie could see it. Peter's skin had become puffy and white, and there were bags under his eyes all the time now; even in the morning. Last month, the computer company he worked for had announced that Peter's plant would be shut down next year. A sick wife and almost no job. Peter was clearly struggling.

"I'm sorry," Julie said now. "I shouldn't have lost my temper."

Peter looked at her. "This is hard, Julie. It's very hard."

"I know," Julie said. "It is hard."

On June 12, Dr. Goldstein's nurse called. Julie's third Adriamycin treatment was scheduled for June 21. The nurse reminded Julie that the twenty-first would be her next-to-last treatment with "Adria." "You have one more session after this; then you go on to the Cytoxan. Cyto's the easy one."

Good, Julie said. She could use something easy.

The next day, Emily called. She was supposed to drive Julie to Fox Chase the next day, but her car was not working. "The transmission," Emily said. "I'm sorry, it just happened this morning. The garage says it won't be ready until Friday. Can Aunt Grace take you?"

But Aunt Grace was in Palm Beach; she and her husband had just bought a new home there.

"Why don't you call Dad?" Emily said. "The Flyers season is over and he's retired. He'll be able to take you."

Julie picked up the phone, dialed the Huntingdon Valley number, and took a deep breath. If Yvonne answered it would be awkward.

"Hello." It was her father. No one said hello like Bob Senior.

Julie explained her predicament. The appointment at Fox Chase was for two, she said. "Can you drive me, Dad?"

"Two. Two works for me, Julie."

The next afternoon, when he picked Julie up at St. Monica's, she told him that Susan had offered to drive her home. "She called last night. You don't have to stay, Dad. You can just drop me off in the parking lot."

But Bob Senior insisted on staying. He sat with Julie through the entire session, except for the times when a nurse came over to check Julie's port, then he would suddenly get thirsty. "Excuse me, Julie," he would say, "I think I'll get a little drink." In between visits to the water fountain, he talked about the weather, his favorite post–hockey season topic.

A few days after the third Adriamycin treatment, the last of Julie's hair fell out.

"I look like a three-minute egg now," she said the next morning at breakfast.

"You look fine," Peter said.

"That's because you haven't seen me bald."

Julie was sleeping in a wig now. The wig, which she'd bought in May, was fine for work, but uncomfortable for sleeping, especially now when the nights were hot. The wig scratched and itched and made Julie's scalp sweat. For a while, she thought about sleeping with nothing, just her bald head, but cancer or no cancer, she was still a thirty-four-year-old woman. Whatever femininity and sexuality she had left, she wanted to keep.

One evening on her way home from work, Julie stopped at a clothing outlet on Route 684 and bought a Philadelphia Phillies cap.

"I think I look kinda cute in it," she said that night. She and Peter were sitting in bed.

Peter told her that she did look cute. But he wanted to go to sleep now. "Take the cap off; I'm going to shut the light off."

"I'm going to wear it to bed," Julie said.

"You can't wear a baseball cap to bed."

"Yes, I can."

"I can't see you in the dark, Julie."

Julie said she didn't care; she was still going to wear the Phillies cap to bed.

Two weeks later, the cap came up again, this time in a conversation with Deidre Newton, Jennifer's oldest daughter.

The day before the Newtons' Philadelphia visit, Rick had called Peter to make a drink date.

"What's the date for?" Julie asked. She was standing on the hall stairs when the phone rang.

Peter shrugged. "Rick says he's learned a lot about doctors and hospitals. He wants to pass it on—you know, help us avoid mistakes."

Around five the following Saturday, a car pulled into the Conte driveway. A moment later, the doorbell rang. Julie, who was sitting in the living room in her Phillies cap, let Peter get the door.

"How was the flight up?" she heard him ask.

"We had some turbulence over Atlanta," someone replied. Rick. Leave it to Rick to notice turbulence over Atlanta.

Julie sensed that someone was staring at her. She turned around. Deidre was standing in the hall.

She pointed to the Phillies cap. "My mommy used to wear a hat like that."

"I know," Julie said.

"Are you bald, too?"

"Uh-huh. Yes," Julie said.

"Do you have a wig?"

"Upstairs." Julie pointed to the ceiling.

Deidre asked what color the wig was.

"Brown, chestnut brown."

"My mommy's wig was blond."

"I know," Julie said.

"Are you sick, too?"

"Yes," Julie said. "I'm sick, too."

Later that evening, when they were alone, Julie asked, "What did you two talk about?" She and Peter were sitting on the living room couch watching the ten o'clock news.

Peter picked up the remote and muted the sound. "Mostly nuts-and-bolts stuff. Rick told me the kinds of questions to ask, what to do if we need a second opinion. Things like that. He wasn't happy with Jennifer's treatment."

Peter put the sound back on. Julie grabbed the remote and muted the TV again. "That's all you talked about? You were gone for nearly three hours."

Peter shrugged. "I think Rick was doing this more for himself than for me."

Peter was probably right about that, Julie thought. She described the exchange with Deidre. "She knew I had cancer right away. As soon as she walked in, she knew. It was the Phillies cap, I think. Jennifer used to wear an Arizona Rangers cap; Deidre must think everyone who wears a baseball cap has cancer."

Peter said it was not the cap. "Rick told her you had cancer."

"Why would Rick do that?" Julie asked.

Peter took the remote out of Julie's hand and put the sound back on. "Why does Rick do anything?" he said.

A few days later, roughhousing on the living room floor, Brittany accidentally knocked Julie's wig off. For a moment, Brittany seemed stunned, but then she began to laugh. It was a great joke, a perfect joke. A bald mother. Who could have imagined?

Julie started to laugh too, but then she thought about the conversation with Deidre.

"C'mon, Mommy." Brittany was tugging at her leg. "Play more." Julie shook her head. "No, not now, hon. Mommy's tired. Mommy will play with you later."

CHAPTER NINE

MORTAL ILLNESS ALWAYS SURPRISES.

No one believes it will happen to her, and when it does, it takes a long time to process the knowledge that you may die.

It took Julie six months to admit the possibility. And there were many times in those months when her mind rebelled against the knowledge, when it insisted that the cancer was a horrible mistake. Winters and Fowble and Goldstein—everyone—had somehow gotten Julie mixed up with another Julie Conte, who also was thirty-four, lived in Newtown, Pennsylvania, had a husband named Peter, two children named Brittany and Mark, and worked at St. Monica's Hospital.

It was almost as if the cancer had anesthetized Julie. Occasionally, a smile from Brittany or a conversation with Peter would puncture the numbness, and Julie would feel a prick of sharp pain. But the prick would only last a moment; then the dull, druglike stupor would envelop her again. Some days, Julie felt as if she were walking under water, others, as if her nerves were sheathed in cement.

In July, however, the anesthetic began to lift. The most palpable sign of change was Julie's reassertion of her autonomy. Almost all her doctors' visits, except the very early ones, had been family affairs. The anesthetized Julie had been too numb to act on her own. Someone, usually Peter or Aunt Grace, was needed to drive her to appointments and to ask questions. But just before the Fourth of July weekend, the newly awakened Julie decided that it was time to change that; she would go to her next appointment at Fox Chase alone.

"You're sure you're up to it?" Aunt Grace asked when she called to offer Julie a ride.

"The appointment's not for chemo," Julie said. "I'm just going for a consultation. I have to see Fowble. I'll be able to drive afterward." Sweet, warm, thoughtful Dr. Fowble was a good doctor to start being autonomous with, Julie thought. She had seen the radiologist alone once already. And the meeting was only an orientation. Nothing scary would be discussed. Dr. Fowble was just going to explain how radiation therapy worked. The trial would end in six weeks and the radiation would begin almost immediately after. It was time for Julie to be briefed on the treatment.

"Why don't I schedule your impression for that day, too," the radiology nurse said when she called Julie to arrange the consultation. "You'll be able to get everything taken care of at once."

Julie asked what an impression was.

"It's sort of like a fitting for a bridge," the nurse said. "You won't feel a thing."

The nurse was half right. A week later, Julie found herself lying nude from the waist up on a metal table with a white foam half-body cast strapped to her back. Julie shifted slightly; the damp, sticky goo inside the cast felt cold against her exposed flesh. "How long do I have to lie like this?" she asked.

The radiology technician looked at his watch, then at Julie. "It takes about ten minutes for the impression to harden."

Julie gazed up at the beam over the table. The technician had aligned it over her left breast before he added a solvent to the goo in the cast. The solvent was supposed to make it harden. "The impression will save you a lot of time," the technician said; he wiped the chemical off his hands. "With the impression, we won't have to fuss around before each treatment. You just strap it on your back, lie on the table, and we'll know exactly where to position the beam."

Julie looked up at the eye again. It almost looked alive in the kind of half-somnolent, half-alert way a snake looks alive. She shifted again. The technician saw her this time. "I'm sorry," he said. "But you can't move. You have to lie . . ."

Julie was not listening anymore. She was wondering how many sessions in a tub of blue goo, how many chemotherapy treatments she would endure for more life. At the start of treatment, she had thought she knew. She would do everything necessary to save her life, but if the cancer came back . . . she would not make herself go through chemotherapy a second time. Jennifer had suffered horribly the second time; Jennifer had paid too high a price for more life.

But now that the anesthesia had lifted, Julie was not so sure. Sometimes, looking at Mark and Brittany, she thought she would be willing to spend the next twenty years chained to a bed of hot coals if it meant that she could see her children graduate from high school and college and start their own lives.

"Finished," the technician said. He was standing over Julie. "You can wash up over there." He pointed to a white door at the opposite side of the room. "There's a washbasin inside."

There was a mirror above the washbasin; as Julie was putting on her blouse, she looked at the port between her breasts. Would Goldstein remove it at the end of the trial? It was funny; in May, Julie had dreaded the start of the trial, but now that it was more than half over, she was dreading its end. After the last three Cytoxan treatments, there would only be six weeks of radiation—and then, nothing. Julie would be defenseless again. Any cancer cells that had survived the drugs and the beam in the other room would be free to do whatever they wanted.

Julie finished buttoning her blouse, then checked her watch. It was nearly eleven. She fussed with her hair for a moment, then picked up her handbag.

When she walked out of the bathroom, the technician was writing something in a notebook. He looked up and smiled. "See you in a few weeks," he said.

"See you in a few weeks," Julie replied.

Dr. Fowble's office was on the other side of the park. Julie went out through the cafeteria onto a walkway. There were only a half dozen people sitting on the grass this morning. Surprising. Usually on warm summer days, the lawn was full of staff and patients. Then Julie remembered, it was only eleven. The park did not fill up until lunchtime.

Dr. Fowble was sitting at her desk under a row of X rays when Julie arrived. The radiologist must have sensed a presence in the doorway. She looked up before Julie had a chance to knock.

"Good morning. How are you?"

Dr. Fowble's alert eyes darted from Julie's face to the empty doorway behind her. "I'm alone today," Julie said.

"No Aunt Grace?"

Julie shook her head. "No Aunt Grace."

Dr. Fowble looked pleased. Grace was smart and supportive and asked good questions, but the radiologist worried about Julie's dependence on her. In Grace's presence, Julie often seemed like a little girl, a helpless little girl. "I thought Julie's decision to come to the consultation alone very significant," Dr. Fowble would say later. "It indicated that she was feeling more secure about herself, that she had stopped being scared. That she could take care of herself now."

Now Julie wanted to talk about her illness. About how much it had frightened her at the beginning and how positive she was starting to feel about it now. "I think that's the most important thing, being positive," Julie told Dr. Fowble. "I think you can't have a healthy body unless you have a positive mind."

"Why do I think you're feeling very positive today, Julie?" Dr. Fowble was smiling at her now.

"Because I am," Julie said.

One evening, a few days later, Lisa called.

"I learned something interesting in the city by the bay," Lisa said. She and Andy had spent the Fourth of July weekend at a medical convention in San Francisco.

Julie was sure that Lisa, the jokester, was setting her up for a one-liner. "Oh, really. What?" Julie liked playing straight man.

"I'm pregnant."

There was a can of Skippy peanut butter on the kitchen counter. Julie put her hand on it and began to screw and unscrew the top.

"Who told you?" No, that was the wrong way to put it. "How do you know?" Julie asked.

"A home pregnancy test. Imagine, a hundred doctors in my hotel, and I have to buy a kit at a drugstore to find out if I'm pregnant."

Julie knew an abortion was out of the question. Lisa and Andy were devout Catholics.

"Have you seen your obstetrician yet?"

"Uh-huh, this morning. She was very encouraging. She told me that she's had pregnant women on chemo before." Lisa paused for a moment. "I guess I get to keep my breasts for a while longer."

Last spring, Lisa had begun talking about getting a prophylactic mastectomy. In June, she had even asked Julie for a DNA sample for a gene test. "I still haven't made up my mind," she told Julie that night, "but you have to have a BRCA test to get the surgery, and the doctors can't do the test without DNA from a family member with the gene."

For some reason, until that moment, it had not occurred to Julie that she was a carrier. But, of course, she must be.

"They just need a little blood," Lisa said. "They get the DNA from the blood."

On that night, Julie had said that she would be happy to help. But now, on this night, there was nothing Julie could say or do to help Lisa.

"How do you feel?" she asked.

"Cosmically, or about the pregnancy?" Lisa said.

"Both."

Lisa suddenly dropped the flippant manner. "Someone up there wants me to have this child, Julie. I feel that. I really do. And Andy does, too."

After she hung up, Julie went out to the backyard. It was a lovely evening, cloudless, except for a thin ribbon of silky pink clouds in the east toward Philadelphia. You could almost taste fall in the air. Peter had put the two new Adirondack chairs under the yard's sturdy old poplar. Julie walked over and sat down in one of them.

When the BRCA gene was discovered the previous fall, Julie had read an article about it in the *Philadelphia Inquirer*. According to the newspaper, in some families, the mutation was a thousand years old. That meant the mutation in Julie's DNA could be older than the country she lived in, older than most of the kings and queens she had read about in school, older than the idea that the earth was round.

And in that time hundreds, thousands of ancestors must have carried it. How many of them had died? No, Julie told herself, she would not think about that tonight; she would not think about all the helpless great-great-great-great grandmothers and aunts and cousins who must have died horrible deaths because of a mutant gene.

She meant what she said to Dr. Fowble about being positive. And Julie, the old college biology major, thought she saw something positive in this. In biology, they teach you that nothing can survive the hurly-burly of evolutionary competition without a comparative advantage; without something that creates a special biological edge. Julie decided that the edge for BRCA families was character. Families like hers survived generation after generation, went on and on despite the mutant gene, because they possessed a special strength and endurance, and because they had a talent for loving one another.

Of course, it occurred to Julie that what she was calling evolution could just be another name for God; comparative advantage, another name for the special mercy He extends to those who suffer greatly.

Whatever the source, Julie believed that the talent for family love was very powerful. It could not save Jennifer or her mother, Kay. But it would save her; Julie was sure of it. It would help her recover, and it would protect Lisa.

Two weeks later, Julie had the first of her three Cytoxan treatments. Emily drove her to Fox Chase.

Julie had been hesitant about asking for the ride. She was trying to be as independent as possible now and Cytoxan was supposed to be the "easy" drug. It was reputed to cause minimal side effects. But the nurse who'd told Julie that was also the nurse who'd told her that the first day of chemo would be easy. Julie decided that she ought to have Emily drive her "just in case." It was a wise decision.

Adriamycin had made Julie sick. But except for one episode in the infusion room, the nausea had decreased gradually. It would begin the day after the treatment and only last thirty-six to forty-eight hours. With Cytoxan, Julie began to feel ill almost immediately. Five minutes into the treatment, she was so nauseated that she had to disconnect the catheter. She stood up and pointed to the wastebasket beside Emily.

"What?" Emily said.

Julie began gesturing frantically at the basket. She was afraid of what would happen if she tried to speak.

Emily picked up the basket. "You want this?" She still looked puzzled.

Julie grabbed the basket and stuck her head into it.

"AAARRRRGGGGGHHHH!"

"Oh God, Julie." Emily turned away. Emily was the squeamish sister.

Around six, Peter was talking to his sister Carol when the doorbell rang. He put the phone down and went to the front door.

Emily and Julie were standing on the steps. Emily looked frantic. Julie, drunk. She was still holding the wastebasket in her hand.

"Are you all right?" Peter asked.

"Uh-uh," Julie said. Then she stuck her head in the basket and vomited again.

Brittany was also concerned about Julie. At the day care center the next evening, Brittany's teacher told Peter that she had been very rambunctious that day. "Actually," the teacher said, "Brittany's been pretty rambunctious for a while. I just wondered . . ." The teacher paused for a moment. "You know, if everything was all right at home."

The day care staff did not know about Julie's illness. Julie was afraid that one of the workers might slip and say something to Brittany. "Julie hasn't been feeling well lately," Peter said.

"Ah, that must be it," the teacher said. "Give her my best, please."

Julie felt guilty when Peter told her about the conversation later that night. "It's not fair. Brittany shouldn't have to go through this. I hope she's not upset with me."

Peter put his hand on Julie's. "Don't be silly. Why would Brittany be upset with you? She's very lucky to have you. We're all lucky to have you."

Peter also was changing. He was more open and affectionate than he had been at the beginning of the summer. Sometimes, Julie thought that, like her, he was finally getting used to the idea of the cancer. Other times, she thought that, after months of trial and error, she had finally learned how to talk to him about the disease. Peter was very good as long as you stuck to specific, concrete topics, like a problem with a doctor or with a treatment. It was the big, amorphous subjects, like Julie's fears and anxieties, that made him withdraw. So lately Julie had been avoiding those topics.

Aunt Grace took Julie to Fox Chase for her second Cytoxan treatment, which went much better than her first. She also went to Julie's follow-up appointment with Dr. Goldstein a few days later. Julie had wanted to go to the follow-up alone, but Aunt Grace was insistent. "It's important that we don't let any mistakes happen to you," she told Julie. Julie took this to be a reference to Jennifer. In the spring, Rick had made it pretty clear to Peter that he thought Jennifer might still be alive if she had been monitored more diligently for metastases. Jennifer had had limited-node involvement, and most women with limited-node involvement usually do not relapse and die within two years, Rick said.

It turned out that relapse—or the danger of it—was what Grace wanted to talk to Dr. Goldstein about. Julie was being monitored for metastases via blood tests and chest X rays. Grace told the oncologist that she thought that was inadequate. "I know with Julie's sister they didn't do a bone scan in time and they missed a lot. I think Julie also should have a bone scan."

Dr. Goldstein tried to be sympathetic. "I understand your concern, Grace," she said, "but a bone scan can't pick up an early micrometas-tasis. It wouldn't be of any use to Julie."

Grace also tried to be sympathetic, but she had already lost one niece, a niece who had died a horrible—and maybe preventable—death. "That's what the doctors said about Julie's sister," she snapped. "They were quite mistaken. Her sister's dead now."

Dr. Goldstein started to say something, then stopped. There was no point in arguing with Grace, she decided. Grace was not mad at Julie's "inadequate" monitoring or at her, Lori Goldstein, or at any of the other things at Fox Chase Grace found to complain about. Grace was angry at God or at fate or at whatever name you give to the force that determines human destiny, angry at it for giving her family the BRCA gene.

Julie's final Cytoxan session was on September 3. This was her last official appointment as a SWOG 9313 patient, and it was uneventful. But, coming out of the infusion room, Julie saw a woman sitting alone in the waiting room. The woman was crying softly. Julie walked over and sat down next to her.

"Today's my first day," the woman said.

"The first time is scary," Julie told her. "After that it gets easier."

The woman asked Julie how long she had been on chemo.

"Three months," Julie said. "But it's over now. Today was my last session. It does end."

The woman nodded. "I'll keep reminding myself of that."

Footsteps. Julie looked up. A nurse was approaching.

"Mrs. Spinelli, we're ready for you now."

The woman put her hand on Julie's arm. "Thank you," she said; then she stood up and followed the nurse into the infusion room.

Julie walked out to the parking lot.

In her mind's eye, she had pictured this moment, her exit from the trial, her resumption of normal life, as being full of drama. There would be a band playing, a line of doctors in white coats waiting to congratulate her, Blessed Catherine and Jennifer hovering above in the summer sky. It would be like the end of a movie. But instead, the moment was like life, ordinary. There were only a couple of puffy cottony clouds in the sky, an elderly woman walking across the parking lot with a cane, and Peter standing by the car waving.

Julie called his name.

EPILOGUE

ONE WARM JULY MORNING TWO YEARS AFTER THE TRIAL ENDED, JULIE awoke to the chirping of birds outside her window, a perfectly blue sky, and a tingle of anticipation. Today, July 15, 1997, was Emily's wedding day. And it was going to be a very grand day, indeed. There would be ushers in black cutaways, bridesmaids (including Julie) in fluffy pink gowns, and a church full of family and friends; and later, there would be bright yellow party tents set out on spacious green lawns and dancing till dawn under Japanese lanterns.

It would be wrong to say that this was the first truly happy moment Julie had had since the end of the trial. As the months, and then the years passed, as Julie began to feel safe again, there had been many such moments. But on this July morning, her happiness was entirely unqualified, entirely uncomplicated. It was the happiness of a woman with a good marriage and two wonderful children, the happiness of a woman who had everything she wanted and was now confident that she would keep it.

Family love had seen Julie through—her recovery had been

complete—and it had seen Lisa through a normal pregnancy and birth, and through the decision not to have a prophylactic mastectomy.

Brittany was still a concern, of course. But Julie felt that, somehow, family love would see Brittany through, too. Julie did not know how yet. But she did know that sometimes you just have to believe, you have to have faith. Breast cancer had taught her that.

AFTERWORD

I TRIED NOT TO THINK ABOUT THE FUTURE WHILE I WAS FOLLOWING Edward and Romy and Julie. But I knew that there was a good chance one of the three would relapse, though I never thought it would be Romy. Her numbers seemed too good. The cure rate for osteosarcoma, 65 percent, is relatively high, and Romy's cell kill count, 100 percent, was astonishing.

I suppose, too, I thought "not Romy," because Romy already had had so much misfortune in her life and because she was a child; it wouldn't be fair if it happened to a child, but it did.

Romy did have one year of normal teenage life in between the trial and her relapse, a year in which she had the experience of first love—a boy named Brian—became the manager of her high school basketball team, and wrote a paper on Shakespeare's sonnets that got an A in sophomore English.

During that year, Romy and I spoke several times on the phone, but except for a brief visit to L.A. in the spring of 1996, I did not see her again until September 17, 1997, when she was on the ninth floor again. Two days earlier, a routine scan had picked up a tumor in her right lung. Romy looked wonderful that afternoon; still summer-tanned and growing quite pretty in an intense, young-poetess kind of way.

Two weeks later, she told me that she had decided to refuse a second round of chemo. More treatment was pointless, she felt; chemo had done nothing for Lotte Kauffman except add to the misery of her final months. Besides, Romy pointed out, her chances of being cured by a second round of treatment were almost as low as the chances of the cancer disappearing on its own.

I was surprised at how angry I got at her.

"If you were my child," I said, "I would make you take the chemo. I'd insist."

"But who would you be doing that for?" she asked. "For me or for you?"

The question stopped me. I cannot conceive of anything more awful than standing by and simply allowing a child, mine or anyone else's, to die. But if the treatment was terrible, the chance of success very low, and the child's suffering already very great, would I have the right to make her submit to more treatment just because I wanted her to fight? Jack and Pam had decided that they did not have that right, and after thinking about Romy's question, I decided that the Hochmans were correct. There are certain decisions no human being can make for another, not even a parent for a child.

The other thing that stays in my mind from that talk was Romy's stoicism; it was a remarkable thing to see, a seventeen-year-old coming to terms so completely with her own death.

Not that Romy doesn't want to live. Oh, she wants to live very badly, indeed; but she knows that the odds are against her and she accepts that, just as she has accepted every other hard fact in her young life. The only thing she wants now is a few months of normal life, life without pain, life with normal breathing, life with Brian.

American medicine is a glory of world science, but the rigor and objectivity that makes it a world glory has to be paid for—sometimes in suffering, and sometimes in death.

Ninety percent of the children in the MIOS control group—the untreated group—would not have relapsed with chemotherapy, and with MTP perhaps Romy and Lotte Kauffman and Daniel Gertz would not have relapsed either.

But without the sacrifices made by the children in the MIOS control group, chemotherapy's effectiveness would not have been established; which means that the thousands of OS kids who have benefited from it would not have, and without an 0133 control group, MTP's ability to help future OS victims could never be conclusively determined.

Is that information worth the suffering the kids in the MIOS control group had to endure? Is it worth Lotte's death, and Daniel's relapse, and now Romy's?

The collective judgment of society is that it is. A few have to suffer in order that the many can be helped. It is the necessary but awful price of medical progress. And while the nature of the price cannot be changed, we can change; we can begin to honor the people who pay it for the rest of us.

In a society full of empty heroes, they are real heroes.

No matter what happens to her now, Romy has already made an enormous contribution. Other children may live because of her sacrifice. How many of us can say that we made that kind of difference with our lives?

Acknowledgments

I OWE A SPECIAL DEBT OF GRATITUDE TO ERIC ROSENTHAL, FORMERLY OF Fox Chase Cancer Center, and Nancy Haberman of Rubenstein Associates. Both provided invaluable assistance at critical points in the writing of this book.

I would also like to thank the following men and women for their help and cooperation.

Edward in Winter: Dr. Roy Gulick and Candy Talcbucon of the AIDS clinical trials unit at Bellevue Hospital in New York City; Drs. Emilio Emini, Ferdinand Massari, and Jeff Chodakewitz of Merck; Mike Watts of Merck; and Virginia Harden and John Bowerbox of the National Institutes of Allergies and Infectious Diseases.

Romy's Knee: Drs. Aaron Rausen and Robin Goodman of New York University Medical Center; Lynn O'Dell of NYU Medical Center; Dr. Eugenie Kleinerman of M.D. Anderson Cancer Center in Houston; Dr. Paul Meyers of Memorial Sloan-Kettering Cancer Center in New York; Dr. Michael Link of Stanford University; Dr. Gregory MacEwen of the University of Wisconsin; and Dr. Ezra Greenspan, professor emeritus of medicine at Mount Sinai Medical School in New York. I would also like to thank Debbie Norberg for allowing me to tell the story of her son, Peter.

Julie and Her Sisters: Drs. Alfred Knudson, Lori Goldstein, and Barbara Fowble of Fox Chase Cancer Center in Philadelphia; Dr. Mary-Claire King of the University of Washington (Seattle); Dr. Mark Skolnick of Myriad Genetics in Salt Lake City; Dr. Francis Collins of the Human Genome Project; Dr. Bernard Fisher of the University of Pittsburgh; Dr. Charles Haskell of UCLA; Dr. C. Kent Osborne of the University of Texas; Drs. Larry Norton and Maria Theodoulu of Memorial Sloan-Kettering Cancer Center; and Dr. William Hryniuk of the University of California at San Diego.

I would also like to thank Ellen Methuen, Janice Dorfman, and Debbie Manzini, who participated in an earlier version of this book; my agent, Ellen Levine, who believed in this project before anyone else; Andrea Bozzelli of Fox Chase for her untiring assistance and good cheer; Dr. Loren Fishman, who answered many of my general medical questions; David Puchkoff and Eileen Stukane, for introducing me to the mysteries of the Internet; my wife, Sheila Weller Kelly, for her warm support and incisive editorial advice; my daughter, Suzanne Kelly-Lyall, project director of the Asia Foundation, for her valued critique; and our son Jonathan Kelly, third baseman for the Fieldston Eagles. Jonathan's youth and exuberance provided a constant and needed reminder that there were other worlds beyond the world this book explores.

I owe my greatest debt, of course, to my three subjects. I thank them for allowing me into their lives at a very difficult moment, for putting up with my often intrusive questions, and most of all, for allowing me to bear witness to their quiet courage and determination. They—and their families—will always be an inspiration to me.